Clinical Management

Blood pressure classification guidelines

Category Systolic blood pressure (SBP) Diastolic blood pressure (DBP)

Normal: < 120 and   < 180

Prehypertension: 120–139   or 80–89

Stage 1 hypertension: 140–159 or 90–99

Stage 2 hypertension: > 160 or > 100

Note: According to the National Heart, Lung, and Blood Institute, 2003, you should not identify hypertension with only one blood pressure reading except when this reading is more than 180/110 or is found along with end-organ harm.

Thrombophlebitis

Assessment and medical attention:
Use a Doppler ultrasound and impedance plethysmography for checking the vessels leading to the heart. Use contrast venography as the ultimate way to find where the problem is and how far it has gone. Medical attention includes raising the legs, working out the legs if inactivity is necessary, compression stockings, and anticoagulation (heparin infusion and Coumadin). In someone with a surface case, raise the legs and use a warm wrapping. If the case is deep, stay in bed and raise the leg(s).

Coronary artery disease

Management:
It is very important to lessen the LDL cholesterol to under 100 mg/dL. This may be done with diet if it is 100–130 mg/dL. If LDL > 130, then drugs are needed. Drugs for this include nicotinic acid, bile acid binding resins, hydroxymethylglutaryl coenzyme A (HMG CoA)

reductase inhibitors, and 1 aspirin every day. The patient can use a beta-blocker to keep angina from occurring. They lessen the myocardial oxygen needs. These drugs include metoprolol or atenolol. These may not be used if the patient has bronchospastic disease, bradydysrhythmia, or heart failure. A calcium-channel blocker stops angina from occurring by lessening the myocardial oxygen needs and starting coronary vasodilation. These include nifedipine, verapamil, or diltiazem. A long-acting nitrate stops angina by starting coronary vasodilation. These include isosorbide dinitrate or sustained-release nitroglycerin.

Congestive heart failure

Medical attention:
Find and manage the reason for the problem. The patient must limit sodium and fluid levels, manage amounts of inactivity and activity, and lose weight when needed. Drugs include angiotensin-converting enzyme (ACE) inhibitors such as captopril, enalapril, or lisinopril. Diuretics include hydrochlorothiazide and furosemide. Beta-adrenergic antagonists include carvedilol, which helps by obstructing too much adrenergic stimulation and is used when ACE inhibitors and diuretics are not working. Inotropic treatment helps if there is a slight or moderate systolic problem (such as digoxin). Neurohormonal antagonists (spironolactone) handle big influences regarding rennin-angiotensin-aldosterone activation. Vasodilators may be used as well as a side treatment. The treatment will depend on the stage of CHF. The stages range from A to B to C to D. Patient education is needed. A doctor should be seen when beginning drug treatment or when medical attention is not working.

Lipid profile

Total cholesterol is best at < 200 mg/dL; HDL > 45mg/dl, LDL < 130 mg/dL; triglycerides < 250 mg/dL. Raised total cholesterol combined with low HDL is a sign of danger for heart disease.

Effect of vitamin K on Coumadin

Someone who is taking Coumadin needs to be educated and told NOT to take a multivitamin since it may prevent the medication from working with too much vitamin K. Vitamin K actually stops the effects of Coumadin. The patient will be eating more leafy green vegetables, and this could also put more vitamin K into the system, which would lessen how well the Coumadin works.

Losartan

Losartan (Cozaar) is an ACE inhibitor, usually used for lowering blood pressure and for congestive heart failure; lessens the conversion of angiotensin I to angiotensin II. It is good as a vasoconstrictor. It also stops aldosterone from being let out. Aldosterone is a hormone from the adrenal cortex that influences blood pressure and saline.

Aldactone

A diuretic that allows the patient to retain potassium. This is a brand name for spirolactone. The patient taking this drug needs to be educated regarding the indications of hyperkalemia. If they experience pain in the legs, more tiredness than normal, moodiness, stomach pain or throwing up, they should get in touch with the medical office.

Beta-blockers

Used to treat high blood pressure; restricts epinephrine. It suppresses the heart rate and contraction (the opposite of an inotropic). Should not be used and could harm a patient if the patient's left ventricle is not working properly, particularly when also linked to right-side malfunction.

Calcium channel blockers

Lower the blood pressure; slows flow of calcium to the lining of the coronary arteries; lessens AV conduction; represses the heart rate. Should not be used and could harm a patient if the patient's left ventricle is not working properly, particularly when also linked to right-side malfunction.

Beta-adrenergic blocking agents:
The use of channel blockers and beta-adrenergic blocking agents (which may be in the body or in the eyes) together could create a problem with low blood pressure. The patient may present symptoms of low blood pressure such as light-headedness or falling.

Verapamil (Calan SR):
This is a calcium-channel blocker drug. Check the patient for lessened vascular resistance in the body. This type of drug lessens the amount of discharge that comes from the sinoatrial node and lessens the conduction velocity that goes through the AV node. It lessens the heart rate. The heart and arteries of the body are relaxed, which creates widened blood vessels and lessens the ability of the heart muscle mass to contract. This is the opposite of inotropic.

Niacin

Niacin (nicotinic acid) is used for lowering cholesterol; can have an outcome of vasodilation and create a problem with orthostatic hypotension. Antihyperlipidemic medications can have a side effect of constipation. The drug works better if it is ingested prior to or during eating.

Ischemic heart disease

Medication:
Drugs used include nitrates, beta-blockers, calcium-channel blockers, and aspirin (unless there is a specific reason that the drug is not a good idea for the particular patient).

Digoxin

Used to be the first-line medication for congestive heart failure. Now it is used for anyone with atrial fibrillation, a form of tachycardia, or left ventricle problems.

Unfavorable side effects

- ACE inhibitors – Coughing (1%–30%), head pain, dizzy feeling.
- Calcium channel blockers – Peripheral swelling and fluid, dizzy feeling, head pain, queasiness, tachycardia.
- Thiazide diuretics – Queasiness, vomiting, loose bowels, dizzy feeling, head pain.
- Beta-blockers – Weakness, impotence, moodiness, and difficulty breathing.
- Digoxin – Vision problems, loose bowels, anorexia, queasiness, and vomiting. In an elderly patient, the most frequently seen side effect is an inability to think clearly.

Hyperuricemia

One adverse effect of taking thiazide is this condition, which is a buildup of uric acid in the blood. Problems with uric acid can lead to flare-up and pain in the toes and feet, or gout. Check the blood with a CBC test prior to starting any medical attention.

Procainamide

Procainamide (trade name: Pronestyl) is used for cardiac dysrhythmias. Anyone taking it needs to be checked for antinuclear antibodies. 80% of patients who take this medication over time have antinuclear antibodies. Of these patients, 20% have a condition that is similar to lupus.

Dyslipidemia

Unless contraindicated, the drug choices include HMG-CoA–reductase inhibitors, cholesterol absorption inhibitors, bile acid sequestrants, niacin, and fibric acid derivatives. If the patient has CAD, an HMG-CoA–reductase inhibitor is the best alternative.

AHA code of behavior for rescue breathing

American Heart Association (AHA) code of behavior for rescue breathing (cardiopulmonary resuscitation) – Do this by opening up the air passage. Angle the patient's head back and raise the chin.

Tuberculosis

To keep someone from getting tuberculosis, there are two choices. One is Bacillus Calmette-Guérin (BCG), a vaccine that is used to avert the condition in someone who does not have it yet. This is not a generally utilized for US citizens. The second is the positive PPD converter, which is isoniazid 300 mg taken by mouth every day for 6–12 months.

Asthma

For continuing management of asthma:
- Anti-inflammatory – Inhaled corticosteroids are the most effective. Alternatives are beclomethasone, triamcinolone, flunisolide, or an oral corticosteroid if the patient has a rigorous condition.
- Sympathomimetic – Loosens the bronchial smooth muscle. A long-acting beta-2 adrenergic agent is utilized together with anti-inflammatory medication and is used to avert bronchospasm that occurs with physical activity. Alternatives are: salmeterol (inhaled), or albuterol (oral; sustained release).

- Antimediator – Inhaled, anti-inflammatory drug used continuously for averting indications of asthma and to avert problems with physical activity or allergies. A 4–6-week test is done to see how much it helps the patient. Alternatives are: cromolyn (nebulizer is favored but it also comes in a metered dose inhaler) and nedocromil (but 20% of patients say the flavor is bad).
- Methylxanthine – Often utilized as an extra measure along with anti-inflammatory medications when there are problems during sleeping. Alternatives are: theophylline (taken by mouth; sustained release; a lot of adverse effects; does have medication interactions) or aminophylline (given into the vein and rarely utilized).
- Leukotriene modifier – new medication for this condition; used as another choice instead of a breathed in corticosteroid when the patient has a mild but ongoing problem with asthma and is at least 12 years old. Alternatives include: zafirlukast (must have an unfilled stomach) and zileuton (but this one creates higher liver enzymes).

<u>Slight case, comes and goes:</u>
The patient will not need to take drugs for asthma on a daily basis. The patient can use a short- acting beta-2 adrenergic agonist to handle indications of asthma. When the drug is utilized 3 or more times a week, the patient may need to have long-term attention for the problem.

<u>Fast-acting drugs:</u>
Fast acting drugs for asthma are used to handle acute problems or worsened symptoms of the condition.
- Short acting beta-2 adrenergic agonist – Medication that is preferred to handle acute problems, worsened symptoms, and to avert E.I.B. The alternatives are: albuterol, bitolterol, pirbuterol, and terbutaline.
- Anticholinergic – the ipratropium bromide can give more gain if utilized together with an inhaled beta-2 adrenergic agonist. It also can be taken by itself in a case where beta-

2 adrenergic agonists are not sitting well with the patient. It is a better treatment for COPD than it is for asthma.
- ⬚Systemic corticosteroid – Used in a moderate to severe worsening of symptoms and to avert the symptoms from getting worse. It is also used to quicken the time it takes to get better and to lessen recurrences. Choices include: methylprednisolone, prednisolone, and prednisone.

Mild, continual case:

Drugs for a slight, yet continual case of asthma include taking one drug per day of:
- Small amount of inhaled corticosteroid (200–500 ug QD) split into 2–4 doses. For example, it could be beclomethasone, 2–4 times to breathe it in b.i.d.).
- Breathed in cromolyn or nedocromil, 2 times to breathe it in t.i.d. or q.i.d.
- Theophylline, sustained-release pill, 10mg/kg QD, may take up to 300 mg at the most for the day; keep watching the theophylline amounts. This is not the favored drug, but it is an alternative.
- Leukotriene modifier – Might be needed.
- Short acting, inhaled beta-2 adrenergic agonist if the patient needs fast-acting help. If this is being utilized every day, the patient will require long-term treatment.

Moderate and continual asthma:
- Moderate amount of inhaled corticosteroid. An example is beclomethasone 500–840 mg QD split into 2–4 times per day.
- Moderate amount of inhaled corticosteroid and a long-acting bronchodilator.
- Fast-acting help in the form of a beta-2 adrenergic agonist. When the patient needs more or when they need to utilize a rescue inhaler every day, long-term medical attention is needed.

Significant and continual asthma:

The patient needs to see an asthma expert and needs to take 2–3 drugs per day. These include:

- High-dose inhaled corticosteroid. Example: beclomethasone more than 840 ug in split amounts QD.
- Long-acting bronchodilator, inhaled or oral beta-2 adrenergic agonist or theophylline.
- Corticosteroid taken by mouth – Try to lessen steroids in the body and keep management of it with a high dose of inhaled steroids.
- Fast-acting beta-2 adrenergic agonist used when necessary for indications of asthma.

<u>Preventative drug for asthma:</u>
If the patient is not having worsened symptoms of asthma, they may use inhaled glucocorticoids. These are anti-inflammatory.

Tuberculosis

The patient needs to see a specialist before starting medical attention.
- If it is a sensitive organism, the choices include isoniazid, taken every day, 5 mg/kg up to 300 mg every day for 2 months and rifampin, every day, 10 mg/kg up to 600 mg/kg every day for 2 months. Pyrazinamide, 15–30 mg/kg up to 2 g every day for 2 months is used. Once the 2 months has passed with the patient taking all 3 of these, use isoniazid and rifampin for 4 months, either every day or 2 times a week in the same amounts.
- If it is a resistant bacillus, then use the following along with the medications listed for a sensitive organism: when isoniazid is not working, use ethambutol in addition to it for the initial 2 months, 15–20 mg/kg for 2 months. Use pyrazinamide, 15–30 mg/kg for 2 months or streptomycin, 15 mg/kg IM.

<u>Adverse effects of drugs:</u>
Before beginning treatment, make sure the patient understands the adverse effects that may occur. Educate them as well regarding potentially toxic effects of these medications.
- Isoniazid – There may be nerve damage that begins in the hands and feet, but this can be avoided by taking pyridoxine every day. There may be hepatitis. The patient may

experience abnormal and heightened sensitivity and an exaggerated immune response. Vitamin B_6 must be given with this drug to avoid issues with optic neuritis.
- Rifampin – Substances from the body and urine can be tinted orange and there may be an orange stain on the patient's contact lenses that will not ever go away. There may also be queasiness and vomiting.
- Pyrazinamide – Liver toxicity and too much uric acid in the blood may occur.
- Ethambutol – The patient may get a high body temperature, rash, and an inflamed optic nerve.
- Streptomycin – The patient may experience harmful effects to organs or to nerves in the ear (which can create problems with hearing and/or balance).

Children:

Use combination treatment of isoniazid (INH), pyrazinamide, and rifampin (Rifadin).

Albuterol inhalers

To do the best job, the inhaler should be used in two puffs. Wait 1 minute between the 2 puffs. This way the first one will be used to open the passage, and then the second will get into the lower respiratory tract more effectively. Using an inhaler incorrectly is a frequently seen reason for treatment failure.

Theophylline

Smoking raises the drug's metabolism. It makes the patient need more than they would need if they did not smoke. Eating a high-protein/low-carbohydrate diet also makes the drug become metabolized faster. This diet also lessens the serum concentration. Serum theophylline levels should be 10–20 ug/mL. If it is more than 20 ug/mL, then it is linked to a toxic outcome. This drug may be used together with cimetidine (Tagamet), but be careful, because this combination may raise the theophylline levels and cause a toxic outcome.

Medication uses

Dextromethorphan: used to manage a cough.

Guaifenesin: expectorant.

Pseudoephedrine: decongestant.

Diphenhydramine: decongestant.

Pulmonary edema

The patient may have shortness of breath that is progressively worse along with weakness and a cough that is getting worse. They will need to go to the hospital and begin oxygen treatment, IV furosemide (Lasix) and morphine. If the patient is identified as someone who could have this condition, they should not be sent home or given an outpatient status.

Drug combinations

<u>Levodopa and isoniazid:</u>
Levodopa (Larodopa) is used for patients with Parkinson's disease. If the patient is also taking vitamin B_6, the drug will not work as well. If the patient also needs to take isoniazid (INH), they will have to take vitamin B_6 to keep from having issues with optic neuritis. Therefore, the drug levodopa may need to be changed in a circumstance where the patient needs both of these medications.

<u>Theophylline and erythromycin-based antibiotics:</u>
Erythromycin can cause theophylline to have lessened metabolism. If the patient needs both, think about using a different antibiotic.

Prednisone

Prednisone (Deltasone) is a corticosteroid; holds back immune reactions so that the patient is actually immunocompromised and is more likely to get an infection. If a patient has to take it regularly, they need to be educated about this and told to get medical help when sickness occurs.

Diabetes mellitus

Pharmacologic agents taken by mouth include:
  Beta-cell stimulants (secretagogues):
- Sulfonylureas – 1st generation works very well and for a long time but there is more danger of hypoglycemia (particularly if the patient is aged). It should not be used for pregnant women, patients with sulfa allergy, gestational or type 1 diabetes, or ketoacidosis. There are not many adverse effects. Be careful if the patient has kidney, liver, or heart problems. Hypoglycemia and increased body weight may occur.
- Meglitinides – Makes the patient have temporary but quick pulse of insulin secretion; Repaglinide is the only option; works quickly, ingest prior to eating.
- D-phenylalanine derivatives – nateglinide; works quickly, use 1–30 minutes prior to eating.

Insulin resistance reducers:
  o Biguanide (Metformin) – 1.5 to 2.5 g QD in split amounts. It raises the peripheral insulin sensitivity and keeps liver gluconeogenesis from occurring; helps the patient lose some weight; better lipid profile despite glycemic action. The adverse effects include gas, loose bowels, and a metal taste that is made better by using it when eating and taking the medication more gradually. Do not use if there is kidney, liver, or advanced heart disease. Do not use if serum creatinine is more than 1.5 u/dL for a man or more than 1.4 u/dL for a woman. Very uncommonly seen are cases of high lactic

acid in the blood. Verify patient records with the pharmacy to see if there are any safety measures.
- Alpha-glucosidase inhibitor – Acarbose and miglitol; lessens postprandial blood glucose. Minimal chance of low blood sugar or gaining weight; does not work as well as sulfonylureas or biguanides. Causes gas, bloat, and loose bowels (but these get better as time goes by).
- Thiazolidinediones (pioglitazone, rosiglitazone) – Use as monotherapy for patients with type 2 diabetes or in combination with insulin, metformin, or a sulfonylurea. Pioglitazone is used 15–45 mg QD. Rosiglitazone is 4–8 mg QD. Check the liver in 2-month increments for the initial year and continue checking habitually after that. There is increased chance of low blood sugar if used with another drug. Can cause postmenopausal ovulation and there is a chance of unplanned pregnancy. Could create chance for congestive heart failure. Chance for adverse reaction to numerous medications. Side effects include upper respiratory infection, sinusitis, head pain, pharyngitis, anemia, and swelling and fluid accumulation.
- Agents used together – Metformin and glyburide; Rosiglitazone and metformin; joined together to keep hepatic gluconeogenesis from occurring; work to provoke beta-cell secretion; create more peripheral insulin sensitivity.
- Angiotensin-converting enzyme (ACE) inhibitor – Use when there is not a reason that this would harm the patient – preferred if the patient also has high blood pressure along with diabetes; works to stop the worsening of kidney malfunction.

Insulin:
Vassal or bolus depending on how long the medication works; suggested intervention for verified or suspected type 1 or gestational diabetes, for type 2 diabetes when dietary and/or medication taken by mouth is not working, when the patient has a lot of anxiety, or if the patient cannot take medications by mouth. Some patients require more than 3 injections each day. These may need to utilize the insulin pump. Getting more body weight and requiring glucose checks more often may complicate things. If the patient has an atypical daily life or an unsteady case, think about utilizing more aggressive medical attention so that the patient can

regulate insulin amounts and check and treat low blood sugar. Begin augmentation if the patient is not able to get their $A_{1c} \leq 7$ by using nutrition, physical activity, and the appropriate oral medications. After the routine is set, the urine and plasma glucose will be assessed by the patient 3–4 times every day as the routine needs (depending on how severe the condition is).

Insulin replacement and augmentation:
- The use of an outside source of insulin does not create a contraindication to insulin and glycemic management.
- It is suggested that replacement medication is needed if there is glucose toxicity where the fasting plasma glucose (FPG) > 250 mg/dL including ketosis, lessened body weight, it is a woman who is carrying a child or is planning on becoming pregnant, or if there is significant sickness, inflection, or heart disease.
- After the routine is set, urine and self-checking plasma glucose should be checked 3–4 times every day according to the routine. The amount needed will lessen if the patient has worsening kidney failure. Management is checked in 3–6-month increments. Look at the glycosylated Hgb to see the average glucose amounts for the prior 8–12 weeks if needed.

Insulin replacement therapy:
Insulin for replacement therapy – For basal bolus insulin, taken with meals; begin by utilizing 0.5 units/kg QD. Think about using a mixed amount of insulin b.i.d. when the patient is very habitual about mealtimes and routines, has a reason to necessitate an easier routine, or has problems affording medication. Normal insulin is not supposed to be more than 50% of insulin that is put into the patient. You should not combine lente or ultralente and regular because the zinc in lente affects it. You should not combine lente and short-acting Velosulin (Nordisk) because of the phosphate buffer. When combining regular and NPH using the identical syringe, draw up the regular earliest. You should not combine glargine and another insulin. You should not utilize a syringe that was utilized for another insulin to draw up glargine.

<u>Insulin augmentation:</u>

Utilized if A_{1c} at or less than 7 with nutrition, physical activity, and insulin taken by mouth. Use 0.14 mg/kg QD for NPH, taken either when the patient goes to bed or twice daily. This amount changes depending on the FPG in order to get glycemic management. The objective is to get the FPG at 80–130 mg/dL. In a case where the FPG is correct and the A_{1c} is >7, and postprandial glucose amounts are ≤ 180 mg/dL, change the patient to replacement medication. Regulate only one insulin medication at one time and change the amount by only 2–5 units. This should be done in 2–3 day increments.

<u>Insulin purity:</u>

- Regular beef/pork – > 10 < 25 parts per million (ppm) proinsulin, which is an immunogenic medication.
- Purified beef/pork – < 10 ppm proinsulin.
- Human synthetic – < 10 ppm proinsulin.
- Beef will have more of an antibody response than pork; human insulin will have the least antibody response.

Hyperthyroidism

- Propranolol, 10–60 mg taken orally in 6-hour increments to handle indications of the condition.
- Radioactive iodine (^{131}I) as the favored medication in the United States; 80–120 mCi in amounts of 5–15 mCi depending on the approximated weight of thyroid gland. The majority get euthyroid when 6–8 weeks have gone by. Hypothyroidism is a common issue and may arise during any stage following ^{131}I. Pregnant women should not use it.
- Antithyroid medication – Used for beginning management of thyrotoxicosis, particularly if the woman is pregnant, the patient does not wish to utilize radioactive iodine, or if the patient is getting ready for an operation. It works for patients who have little goiters. Propylthiouracil (PTU) is 300–400 mg QD in split amounts and is favored in pregnancy. For a pregnant woman, use less than 200 mg QD. Methimazole (MMI) is

15–60 mg every day taken by mouth in 3 split amounts. Adverse effects include skin inflammation, queasiness, agranulocytosis, or hypothyroidism that can create a TSH-provoked enlargement of the goiter.

Adult hypothyroidism:
- The average substitution amount of T_4 will be thyroxine, 0.125 mg/day for an otherwise well, fully grown patient who is not aged. This can be 0.25–0.3 mg each day.
- Begin the dose by using 0.1 mg every day if the patient has not turned 50 yet. Use 0.025 for someone that is 50 or older and has an identified ischemic heart disease but not angina.
- Raise the amount in 0.025 mg increments per day every 2 weeks pending the patient becoming euthyroid.
- If there is also adrenal inadequacy, heart inadequacy or angina, special management will be needed.
- The beginning results will generally not be obvious until a minimum of 2 weeks has gone by. Signs that the medicine is working begin with lessened swelling and fluid in the face and more urine.

Laboratory values:

Assessments to identify category of hypothyroidism:

Category	TSH	FT_4	FT_3
Primary hypothyroidism	raised	lowered	lowered
Subclinical hypothyroidism	raised	normal	normal
Secondary, with pituitary deficiency	lowered	lowered	lowered

Where:

TSH – thyroid stimulating hormone

FT₄ – thyroxine

FT₃ - triiodothyronine

Thyroid nodule

Medical attention:

Cut out the nodule and localized lymph nodes as needed. Total thyroidectomy may be needed for someone with medullary carcinoma. Get rid of metastasis by utilizing big amounts of radioactive iodine. Hold back the work of the thyroid by using L-thyroxine. Utilize chemotherapy if the condition is anaplastic carcinoma. Holding back thyroid work and using radioactivity to get rid of metastasis will not work in a case of medullary thyroid carcinoma.

Cushing's syndrome

Medication therapy:

If the patient cannot have an operation for it, uses radiation and medication. Drugs are ketoconazole, 400–500 mg b.i.d., metyrapone, 2 g every day, and aminoglutethimide, 1 g each day.

Addison's disease

Medication therapy:

Use cortisol, 15–20 mg taken by mouth each morning, then 5–10 mg between 4:00 and 6:00 in the evening. Use fludrocortisone acetate, 0.05–0.3 mg every day or on alternate days when there is inadequate sodium being kept into the body from using cortisol by itself.

Dysmetabolic syndrome

According to the National Cholesterol Education Program (NCEP) Adult Treatment Panel (ATP) III standards regarding identifying dysmetabolic syndrome, the patient has the condition if 3 of these are true:
- Triglyceride > 150 mg/dL.
- High-density lipoprotein (HDL) cholesterol is < 40 mg/dL for a male or < 50 mg/dL for a woman.
- Measurement of the waist is more than 102 cm (40 inches) for a male or more than 88 cm (35 inches) for a female.
- Blood pressure – 130/85 mm Hg.
- Fasting glucose is more than 110 mg/dL.

Glargine

Glargine (Lantus) is a long-acting background insulin. It is generally used one time each day. Glargine came onto the market in 2001. Generally it is believed that is works for 24 hours and has no peak. It is transparent. It has to be used by itself and cannot be used in combination with another form of insulin.

Common prescriptions

Humalog (Lispro): Generally used 3 times QD and taken during mealtime.

Nova log (Aspart): Generally used 3 times QD and taken during mealtime.

Glipizide

In Glipizide (Glucotrol), Sulfonylureas lessen the patient's blood glucose by provoking insulin to come out of the pancreas. As time goes by, it could essentially raise the insulin outcome on a cellular level and lessen the amount of glucose created in the liver. This type of drug is utilized for someone that has a normal pancreas and type 2 diabetes.

Insulin pump

Patients frequently object to skin and area difficulty that have to do with the dressing bonding agent not attaching or red skin and pain on the area. It is a common cause for a patient to stop using an insulin pump. Other concerns are time and expense. In defense of the insulin pump, the 1993 Diabetes Control and Complications Trial (DCCT) showed that using the insulin pump and a number of injections done every day gave the patient less of a chance for microvascular difficulties.

Pioglitazone

Pioglitazone (Actos) or rosiglitazone (Avandia) are used to treat patients who have gestational diabetes. They raise the glucose uptake that goes into the muscle and fat. Patients with gestational diabetes need insulin. They do not need an insulin sensitizer.

Desmopressin acetate

Side effects include water intoxication, which causes the patient to have lassitude, alteration in how he acts, confusion, or show signs of neuromuscular excitability. The purpose of this drug is to help water reabsorb into the renal tubules.

Insulin injections

<u>Children:</u>
2:1 proportion NPH/regular for the morning. 1:1 each evening. Alter it depending on the blood sugar. Check blood sugar 4 times every day. The amount is determined by times of insulin activity.

Lispro

Lispro (Humalog) is a first analog of human insulin. Benefits are that it works faster and lasts for a shorter time. It gets to peak in 1–2 hours and lasts for 4 hours. Regular insulin lasts for 6–8 hours. It is handy for some patients because it can be used just 10–15 minutes before a meal. It has been available since June 1996, so there is not a long-term safety profile yet. The effects on a fetus are not known. It costs more than insulin. Some insurance companies do not pay for this medication.

Sulfonylurea treatment

Frequently seen adverse outcomes include hypoglycemia or more body weight.

Headaches

Management:

Tension headache: Use an analgesic (no prescription necessary), e.g.:
- Acetaminophen, 650–1000 mg q.i.d.
- Aspirin, 650–1000 mg q.i.d.
- Ibuprofen, 400 mg q.i.d.

If these do not work, try an antimigraine agent.

Cluster headaches:
- Ergotamine tartrate, 2 mg daily, 0.5–1.0 mg per rectum or 0.25 mg SQ t.i.d. for 5 days in the week.
- Prednisone, 20–40 mg every day or q.o.d. lasting 2 weeks; gradually stop using this medication.
- Verapamil, 240–480 mg daily.
- Methysergide, 4–6 mg daily.

If the cluster headache is acute:
- Medication taken by mouth does not generally work.

- Sumatriptan, 6 mg SQ.
- Ergotamine tartrate inhaled aerosol – Works for some patients.
- 100% inhaled oxygen – Generally works if the patient has cluster headache.

Migraine headache:
- Aspirin, 650–1950 mg every day.
- Propranolol, 10-20 mg b.i.d. to begin with, and then using more each time to get to 80–120 mg every day. This should not be used if the patient has congestive heart failure, blocking lung disease, diabetes or significant depression.
- Amitriptyline, 10–150 mg every day – Another tricyclic antidepressant may be useful; use for 2–4 weeks before results are noticed. Do not use if there is cardiac dysrhythmia, narrow angle glaucoma, or a problem with urination.
- Selective serotonin reuptake inhibitors (SSRIs) – Preferred if the patient is elderly or has a heart condition. Frequently used are fluoxetine, sertraline, paroxetine and venlafaxine. Begin with 10 mg each day at 7 in the morning. Move up to 20 mg within 7 to 10 days of use. Do not use if the patient has significant depression.
- Calcium-channel blockers – Used a lot, but these do not work as well as the other alternatives. Use verapamil, 40 mg t.i.d. to start, then titrate up to 80 mg t.i.d. in the next 2–3 weeks. The most you can take of this is 160 mg t.i.d. Do not use if the patient has congestive heart failure, heart obstruction, or low blood pressure.

Acute migraine headache: Lie back somewhere that has no sound or light, use a simple analgesic (aspirin) right when it starts to ease the pain somewhat. Medicines that may be used include:
- Nonsteroids – Naproxen, 250 mg used every 1–4 hours as necessary; ketorolac, 10 mg every 1–4 hours as necessary.
- Drugs that have butalbital in them – Aspirin/caffeine/butalbital together; acetaminophen/caffeine/butalbital together.

- Opiate – Can work but prudence is necessary for this drug. Butorphanol, 1 mg in 4-hour increments; Meperidine, 75–100 mg including hydroxyzine 50 mg in 4-hour increments.
- Selective serotonin reuptake inhibitors – A number of varieties may be used. Do not use if the patient has coronary artery disease, Prinzmetal's angina, basilar and hemiplegic migraine, high blood pressure that is not being managed, past anaphylaxis, or lately utilized ergotamine.
- Ergot alkaloid – Taken orally or by suppository. Do not use if the patient is pregnant, or has high blood pressure that is not being managed, peripheral vascular disease, coronary artery disease, or liver or kidney problems. Avoid simultaneous utilization of sumatriptan.
- Migranal, 2-mg nasal spray.
- Drugs for queasiness as necessary.
- Acetaminophen, aspirin and caffeine – taken orally.

Transient ischemic attack

When the cardiac emboli are likely, do quick anticoagulation with IV heparin and then oral warfarin sodium. Use aspirin, 325 mg daily if cardiac emboli are not as likely. If the patient cannot use aspirin, use platelet inhibitors, such as:
- Dipyridamole/ASA, 50 mg daily if the patient has prior TIA or CVA during a time of using aspirin.
- Clopidogrel bisulfate, 75 mg if the patient is allergic to aspirin or cannot use aspirin for another reason. Be careful with this medication if there is significant liver disease.
- Ticlopidine, 250 mg b.i.d. if the patient is not able to use the other alternatives. Continue to check for neutropenia or agranulocytosis.

Only use carotid thromboendarterectomy if the arteriogram shows that more than 70% of the stenosis can be affected by an operation, there is minimal atherosclerosis elsewhere, and the patient adequately qualifies for the operation.

Acute seizure disorder

Management:

Diazepam, 5–10 mg in a slow IV; lorazepam, 4 mg in a slow IV. Do not use medicine if the patient has alcohol withdrawal seizures.

Prevention:
- Manage conditions underneath the seizure as needed (infections or metabolic problems).
- Use medication appropriate for the type of seizure.
- Tonic-clonic or partial – Use phenytoin, 200–400 mg every day or split in two, and keep the serum level up to 10–20 ug/mL. Phenytoin cannot be used if the patient has sinoatrial or atrioventricular obstruction. Use carbamazepine, 600–1200 mg daily, split into two, and maintain the serum at 4–12 ug/mL. Do not use carbamazepine if there is a problem with tricyclic antidepressants, the patient has had or is having a bone marrow depression, or the patient is taking monoamine oxidase inhibitors.
- Valproic acid, 1500–2000 mg, split into three times a day, and maintain serum at 50–100 ug/mL (not for anyone who has hepatic disease).

Seizures

Petit mal:
- Ethosuximide, 100–1500 mg, split into two times a day, but be very careful of this medication if the patient has hepatic or renal disease.
- Valproic acid, in same amounts as for tonic-clonic.
- Clonazepam, 0.05–0.2 mg/kg, split into two times a day, and maintain serum level at 20–80 ng/mL. Do not use clonazepam if the patient has a problem with benzodiazepines, hepatic disease, ongoing breathing problems, or glaucoma that is not being managed medically.

<u>Myoclonic seizure:</u>
- Valproic acid in the same amounts as with tonic-clonic.
- Clonazepam in the same amounts as petit mal.

<u>Partial or secondary generalized seizure:</u>

These antiseizure drugs used for adjunctive treatment have not been available for as long as some others:
- Gabapentin, 900–1800 mg each day, split into two times a day.
- Lamotrigine, 100–500 mg each day, split into two times a day.
- Topiramate, 200–400 mg each day, split into two times a day.

Parkinson's disease

Levodopa/carbidopa, 25/100 or use sustained release in 50/200 t.i.d. as the beginning medication that is favored more than others in a case that is worsening more quickly. This will help every clinical element but will not stop the worsening. Do not use if the patient has narrow-angle glaucoma, a psychiatric problem, or is already utilizing MAOIs. Be careful with this medication if there is malignant melanoma or an active ulcer.

<u>Dopamine agonists:</u>
Provoke the dopamine receptors (in brain) and can be utilized as monotherapy in the initial stages or in combination with levodopa/carbidopa. Choices include:
- Ropinirole, 0.25–3 mg t.i.d., but the side effects are decrease in blood pressure upon standing, syncope, and hallucination.
- Pramipexole, 1.5–6 mg q.d., but the side effects are decrease in blood pressure upon standing, hallucination, somnolence, queasiness, and vomiting.
- Bromocriptine, 1.25 mg b.i.d. and then up titrate until the indications improve. Do not use if the patient has had psychiatric problems, heart attack, peripheral blood vessel disease, or bleeding ulcer.

Catechol-o-methyl transferase (COMT) inhibitors:
Assists levodopa/carbidopa. Tolcapone is used 100–200 mg t.i.d. Maximum dose of entacapone is 200 mg for every time levodopa/carbidopa is used, up to 1600 mg q.d. Be careful of this medication if the patient has liver disease. Stop using tolcapone in 3 weeks if there is not a clinical reaction because of the danger of hepatocellular harm.

Selegiline:
Use 5 mg b.i.d., in combination with levodopa, taken with the first and second meal of the day. The reaction is not the same for all patients. Proof that it stops the condition from worsening necessitates that this medication be well thought out for anyone with the condition in a slight or early stage.

Amantadine:
Use 100 mg b.i.d., but the way it works is not known. It does help indications if the condition is slight. Adverse outcomes are bewilderment, depression, fidgeting, low blood pressure, and heart irregularities have occurred in some patients.

Anticholinergics:
Ease spasm and stiffness. Use benztropine mesylate, 1–6 mg daily. Use trihexyphenidyl, 6–20 mg every day. This medication is not well accepted by an elderly patient. Potential adverse outcomes include not being able to urinate as often, more pressure inside the eye, irregular heart rhythm, and infrequent and difficult stools. Do not use if the patient has narrow-angle glaucoma, enlarged prostate gland, or a blocking gastrointestinal condition.

Clozapine:
Use 6.25 mg, and up titrate to 25–100 mg. This medication is used to help bewilderment, psychosis, and involuntary and sometimes extreme movements. Continue to monitor CBC.

Therapy:
The patient may need speech or physical therapy.

Operation:

Thalamotomy or pallidotomy may be considered as an option if the patient has a significant case and cannot take the drugs to help the situation.

Post-herpetic neuralgia

Anticonvulsants, tricyclic antidepressants, and opioids.

Peripheral vestibulopathy

Use a scopolamine patch in back of the ear for a duration of 3 days. Use meclizine (Antivert), 12.5 mg–25 mg PO t.i.d. to q.i.d. Use dimenhydrinate (Dramamine), 50 mg t.i.d. or q.i.d. Use Compazine, 5 mg–10 mg q4h prn.

Adverse effects

Phenytoin (Dilantin):

Frequent adverse effect is hyperplasia of the gums. The patient needs to practice proper and habitual care of the mouth and teeth.

Sinemet:

Used for Parkinson's disease, can cause low blood pressure, stomach upset, psychosis, and problems with motor skills. Do not take with meals even though there are gastrointestinal problems because it absorbs into the body better without food. It does not slow down the worsening of Parkinson's disease.

Trigeminal neuralgia

These drugs might begin to work and help the indications in approximately 24 hours, but generally they start to work in 4–6 hours. Check the blood levels when needed (contingent upon how much of the drug is going to be used). The patient can use drugs to handle seizures.

HIV

Antiretroviral therapy:
Medication choices alter quickly, so check with an expert in the field. According to the CDC from 2002, the favored medication is highly active antiretroviral therapy, or HAART. The use of antiretroviral medication is contingent on how quickly the condition is worsening.

- First choice – For a patient who has $CD4^+$ count of less than 500 or viral RNA levels more than 5000. This is the main concern when choosing when to begin treatment.
- Second choice – For a patient who has detectable plasma viral RNA that is > 500 without concern for what the $CD4^+$ count is or what the clinical stage is.
- Third choice – For any patient who is HIV positive, regardless of viral RNA being negative and $CD4^+$ count being more than 500.

Medication needs to be started for anyone with indications of HIV, such as perspiration during sleeping or yeast infections that come back time and again.

Antiretroviral medications:
- Nucleoside reverse transcriptase inhibitors (NRTs) include: zidovudine (AZT) may cause anemia, head pain, queasiness and muscle soreness. Stavudine (d4T) may cause peripheral abnormal nerve functioning. Didanosine (ddl) may cause pancreatic, loose stools, and peripheral abnormal nerve functioning. Zalcitabine (ddC) may cause mouth ulcers, peripheral abnormal nerve functioning and pancreatic. Lamivudine (3TC) may cause queasiness and head pain.

- Non-nucleoside reverse transcriptase inhibitors (NNRTI) – nevirapine may cause skin irritation. Delavirdine may cause skin irritation. Efavirenz may cause vertigo, bewilderment, and sleepiness.

Protease inhibitors (PI):

Saquinavir may cause loose stools, queasiness, and head pain. Indinavir may cause kidney stones and too much bilirubin. Ritonavir may cause problems with other medications and it has an astringent taste following taking it. Nelfinavir may cause loose stools and raised liver function assessment (LFT). Amprenavir may cause stomach problems. Lopinavir may cause stomach problems or high cholesterol.

Viral load:

Check the viral RNA in increments of 3–4 months. Check it more often when you think the patient may not be taking medications properly, the $CD4^+$ count goes down, clinical indications show up, or when alterations in medication become necessary (in which case you should check in 4–8 weeks and check again in 3–4 weeks to make sure the medication is working as it should).

Beginning medication:

Be sure the patient is taking the medication as it is supposed to be taken. Difficult routines are very hard to stick to. Viral replication will be faster and happen right away when the medication is not taken properly.

HAART:

HAART medication is the use of 3 or more HIV medications used together. These combinations may be: Efavirenz along with 2 nucleoside/nucleotide reverse transcriptase inhibitors; indinavir along with 2 NRTIs; nelfinavir along with two NRTIs; ritonavir and indinavir along with 2 NRTIs; ritonavir and lopinavir along with 2 NRTIs; ritonavir and saquinavir along with 2 NRTIs.

Prevention medication:

Prevention medication for opportunistic infections associated with HIV:

- *P. carinii* pneumonia prevention should begin if the CD4$^+$ count is less than 200. Use trimethoprim-sulfamethoxazole (TMP/SMX), 1 double potency pill every day or three times in a week. Use dapsone, 100 mg every day or aerosolized pentamidine, 300 mg every month when the patient cannot use TMP/SMX.
- *Mycobacterium tuberculosis* – use isoniazid, 10 mg/kg every day with a maximum of 300 mg along with pyridoxine, 5- mg every day. Use this for a year. If the patient has a positive PPD response that is 5 mm of induration or more and the chest radiograph is negative, use prevention medication.
- Toxoplasmosis – start if the CD4$^+$ is less than 100. Use TMP/SMX, one double potency pill taken three times a week or every day.
- *Mycobacterium avium* complex – start prevention if the CD4$^+$ count is less than 50. Use clarithromycin, 500 mg taken by mouth b.i.d. OR azithromycin, 500 mg taken by mouth three times a week OR rifabutin, 150 mg taken by mouth b.i.d.

Uncomplicated gonococcal infection

Cervix, urethra and rectum:

Use cefixime, 400 mg taken by mouth in one dose; ceftriaxone 125 mg IM used in one dose; ciprofloxacin, 500 mg taken by mouth in one dose; ofloxacin, 400 mg taken by mouth in one dose; levofloxacin, 250 mg taken by mouth in one dose, PLUS azithromycin, 1 g taken by mouth in one dose or doxycycline, 100 mg taken by mouth two times every day for a week when chlamydial infection could also be part of the condition.

Other choices for this condition include spectinomycin, 2 gm IM in one dose, ceftizoxime, 500 mg IM in one dose, cefoxitin, 2 g IM in one dose together with probenecid, 1 g taken by mouth or cefotaxime, 500 mg IM in one dose or gatifloxacin, 400 mg taken by mouth or norfloxacin, 800 mg taken by mouth, PLUS azithromycin, 1 g taken by mouth in one dose or doxycycline,

100 mg taken by mouth two times a day for a week when chlamydial infection could also be part of the condition.

Pharynx:

Ceftriaxone, 125 mg IM taken in one dose or ciprofloxacin, 500 mg taken orally in one dose, PLUS azithromycin, 1 g taken orally in one dose or doxycycline, 100 mg taken by mouth b.i.d. for a week when chlamydial infection could also be part of the condition.

Pregnant women:

Use an advised or varied cephalosporin. You may use spectinomycin, 2 g in one dose of IM PLUS erythromycin base, 500 mg taken by mouth 3 times every day for a week when chlamydial infection could be or is a part of the condition. Do not use quinolones or tetracyclines.

Genital chlamydial infection

The advised routine is azithromycin, 1 g taken orally in one dose OR doxycycline, 100 mg taken orally b.i.d. for one week. Another option is erythromycin base, 500 mg taken orally q.i.d. every day for a week OR erythromycin ethylsuccinate, 800 mg taken orally q.i.d. every day for a week OR ofloxacin, 300 mg taken by mouth two times a day for a week OR levofloxacin, 500 mg taken by mouth for a week. If it is a pregnant woman, use erythromycin base 500 mg taken by mouth t.i.d. every day for a week. Another option for a pregnant woman is erythromycin base 250 mg taken orally q.i.d. every day for 2 weeks OR erythromycin ethylsuccinate, 800 mg taken orally q.i.d. for a week OR erythromycin ethylsuccinate, 400 mg taken orally q.i.d. for 2 weeks OR azithromycin, 1 g taken by mouth in one dose.

Syphilis

A pregnant woman who is also allergic to penicillin needs to utilize penicillin following desensitization in every phase. Penicillin is the other medical choice for any phase of syphilis other than neurosyphilis. If the case is early and the patient got it in the past 90 days, medically manage every partner. The initial treatment is benzathine penicillin G, 2.4 million units IM one time. If there is a penicillin allergy, use doxycycline, 100 mg taken by mouth b.i.d. for 14 days OR tetracycline, 500 mg taken by mouth q.i.d. for 14 days. For a latent case that has gone on for a while, use benzathine penicillin G, 2.4 million units IM every week for 3 weeks. If allergic to penicillin, use doxycycline, 100 mg taken by mouth b.i.d for 4 weeks OR tetracycline, 500 mg taken by mouth q.i.d. for 4 weeks.

Neurosyphilis

Use 18–24 million units of aqueous crystalline penicillin G every day. This is given in the form of 3–4 million units into the vein in increments of 4 hours. Do this for 10–14 days. If you are sure that the patient will finish the regimen, the other choice for neurosyphilis is 2.4 million units of procaine penicillin IM every day together with probenecid, 500 mg taken by mouth q.i.d. Both of these are used for 10–14 days.

Herpes genitalis

Handle indications as needed with medicines to dry and make the itching better. Use chemotherapeutic agents on the skin, by mouth or by IV. These include acyclovir, famciclovir and valacyclovir. On the skin, medicine has limited use unless the patient has an immune system problem. IV medicine is useful for a significant case or if the patient has a complexity that means he needs to go to the hospital. Since acyclovir comes out with the kidney function, drink plenty of fluids. The use of medication is not thoroughly researched for pregnant women.

Genital warts

If the problem is little and in the vulva or perianal area, the patient can medicate using:

- Podofilox 0.5% solution or gel. Put it on utilizing a cotton tip b.i.d. for 3 days, and then do nothing for 4 days. This routine may be done up to 4 times. Be careful with podophyllin utilization with regard to the dimension of the region being medicated.
- Use 80%–90% solution of trichloroacetic acid (TCA) or herb extract of podophyllin every week for 6 weeks. The patient has to rinse it off when four hours have gone by, and shield the rest of the skin utilizing petroleum jelly.
- The favored method is TCA because it works the best, does not get soaked up and may be utilized for a pregnant woman or on a penis. It does hurt a bit more than podophyllin, but using sodium bicarbonate right away can lessen the pain.
- Imiquimod 5% cream just before going to sleep 3 times a week for 16 weeks. Rinse the area 6–10 hours following application.
- An operation utilizing tangential scissor or shave cut, curettage, or electrosurgery.
- Intralesional interferon.
- Freezing the area utilizing liquid nitrogen.

Bigger warts are defined as being > 2 cm. For utilization on bigger warts or warts on vulva or vagina:
- Utilize CO_2 laser.
- Use electrosurgery to destroy the tissue.
- Use heat to destroy the tissue.
- Destroy the tissue by freezing it.
- Leep.
- Intralesional interferon.

Pelvic inflammatory disease

If the patient is being medically treated from home (as opposed to the hospital), the advisable routine is ofloxacin, 400 mg taken orally b.i.d. for two weeks OR levofloxacin, 500 mg taken orally daily for two weeks together or apart from metronidazole, 500 mg taken orally b.i.d. for 2 weeks. Another choice is ceftriaxone, 250 mg IM used in one dose OR cefoxitin 2 g IM taken in one dose and probenecid, 1 g taken orally at the same time in one dose. Also other parenteral third-generation cephalosporins may be used along with doxycycline, 100 mg taken orally b.i.d. for 2 weeks together or apart from metronidazole, 500 mg taken orally b.i.d. for 2 weeks. Check the patient again in 72 hours. Check again to assess whether the condition has gotten better in 4–6 weeks following medical management. Assess and medically manage anyone who has had exposure.

Vulvovaginitis

Trichomoniasis:
For trichomoniasis, the preferential method is metronidazole, 2 g taken orally in one dose. Another choice is metronidazole, 500 mg b.i.d. for a week. All sexual partners should be given medical attention as well.

Bacterial vaginosis:
For bacterial vaginosis, the preferential method is clindamycin cream, 2% in a full applicator, 5 g put into the vagina before going to sleep for a week. You may use metronidazole, 500 mg taken orally b.i.d. for a week OR metronidazole gel, 0.75% in a full applicator of 5 g put into the vagina q.d. or b.i.d. for 5 days. Another choice is to use clindamycin, 300 mg taken orally b.i.d. for a week (may be used when pregnant), metronidazole, 2 g taken by mouth in one dose, and clindamycin ovules, 100 g put into the vagina before going to sleep for 3 days. If the woman is pregnant, use metronidazole, 250 g taken orally 3 times every day for a week and clindamycin, 300 mg taken orally b.i.d. for a week.

Vulvovaginal candidiasis

Uncomplicated vulvovaginal candidiasis:
Medicine put into the vagina may be butoconazole, 2% cream (5g) for 3 days OR butoconazole, 2% cream (5g) in one application OR clotrimazole 1% (5g) for 1–2 weeks OR clotrimazole, 100 mg in a tablet form (use b.i.d. for three days) OR clotrimazole, 500 in tablet

form (use a single application) OR miconazole, 2% cream (5g) for a week OR miconazole, 100 mg in suppository form (q.d. for a week) OR miconazole, 200 mg in suppository form (one a day for 3 days) OR nyastin, 100,000 unit tablet (one a day for 2 weeks) Ortioconazole, 6.5% ointment (5g) for one application OR terconazole, 0.4% cream (5g) for a week OR terconazole, 0.8% for 3 days OR terconazole, 80 mg in suppository form (q.d. for 3 days).

Creams or suppositories utilized inside the vagina will be made with oil and can make a latex condom or diaphragm become less strong than it normally would be.

By mouth, use fluconazole, 150 mg in a tablet that is taken one time for one dose. The patient should come back for another check-up if the indications come back again within 2 months.

Complicated vulvovaginal candidiasis:
- The preferential method for a reappearing case is one to two weeks utilizing topical azole treatment or fluconazole, 150 mg by mouth repeated after 3 days time. The safeguarding routine may be clotrimazole, 500 mg in suppository form used once a week OR ketoconazole, 100 mg used every day OR fluconazole, 100–150 mg used once a month or 100 mg every day. Safeguarding routines generally go on for 6 months. Patients getting ongoing medication utilizing ketoconazole need to be watched for hepatic toxicity.
- Significant VVC needs 1–2 weeks of topical azole or 150 mg utilizing fluconazole in two doses, one 72 hours after the other.
- Non-albicans VVC needs one to two weeks of medical attention utilizing non-fluconazole azole. When it reappears, use 600 mg of boric acid in a gelatin capsule form, put into the vagina one time a day for 14 days. This patient needs to see an expert.
- If the patient is pregnant, use topical azole medical attention in the vagina for a week.

Urinary tract infection

For a one-dose routine, use fosfomycin tromethamine (3g). A 3-day routine can be used for uncomplicated lower tract infection, including TMP/SMX DS pill b.i.d., ciprofloxacin, 250 mg b.i.d., norfloxacin, 400 mg b.i.d., ofloxacin, 200 mg b.i.d., and levofloxacin, 250 mg every day. For a routine that lasts 7–10 days, which generally is utilized in a complicated lower tract infection, the medicine is TMP/SMX, one DS pill b.i.d., nitrofurantoin, 100 mg q.i.d., trimethoprim, 100 mg b.i.d., norfloxacin, 400 mg b.i.d., ciprofloxacin, 250–500 mg b.i.d., and levofloxacin, 250 mg every day. If the patient is pregnant, use nitrofurantoin, 100 mg b.i.d. for 7–10 days. Another choice is amoxicillin, 500 mg taken orally t.i.d. for 1–2 weeks or cephalosporin, 500 mg q.i.d. for 1–2 weeks. For anyone, think about also using phenazopyridine hydrochloride, 200 mg taken by mouth t.i.d. for 2 days to ease soreness. If you do use this, make sure the patient knows that the urine will turn orange or red.

Acute pyelonephritis

The patient will need to be in the hospital when pregnant, presenting with another condition underneath this one, when there is lessened renal reserve, or if the patient is significantly toxic or cannot use medicine taken by mouth. Significant toxicity is indicated by high body temperature, abnormally low blood pressure, or other symptoms. In the hospital, the patient will need parenteral antibiotics. The IV for antimicrobial treatment will depend upon the results of the culture and sensitivity assessments. The patient will also need to be hydrated with an IV. If the patient does not need to go to the hospital, make sure they will complete the routine and adhere to the treatment. The patient will need to be able to get to the hospital if the indications progress. Antibiotics might include trimethoprim-sulfamethoxazole, first generation cephalosporins, amoxicillin/clavulanate, fluoroquinolones, or ciprofloxacin. 30% of patients are resistant to ampicillin, and therefore it should only be used in combination. Check back with the patient in 24 hours, and drink lots of water.

Acute bacterial prostatitis

Patients who may be septic and/or be unable to void all of the urine need to go to the hospital. If the patient can be treated at home, the best alternative for someone older than 35 years old will be trimethoprim/sulfamethoxazole in a double-strength pill b.i.d. for 2–4 weeks. If the patient is not yet 35 years old, use doxycycline, 100 mg taken by mouth b.i.d. for 10 days along with ceftriaxone, 250 mg IM used once OR ofloxacin, 400 mg one time followed by 300 mg b.i.d. for a duration of 2–4 weeks. The patient will need to be confined to bed. Use sitz bath t.i.d for half an hour. The patient should come back for another check-up in 48 to 72 hours.

Chronic bacterial prostatitis

This condition is commonly hard to manage. The common antibiotics used include trimethoprim/sulfamethoxazole, doxycycline, ciprofloxacin, levofloxacin, and norfloxacin. Antibiotics are used for 4–12 weeks. Advise the patient to stay away from over-the-counter decongestants when there are urinary outlet problems.

Epididymitis

<u>Men younger than 35:</u>
If the patient does not need to go to the hospital and can be treated at home, use antibiotics, depending upon how old the patient is and what the indications are. If the patient is fully grown but less than 35 years old, the preferred medicine is ceftriaxone, 250 mg IM taken in one dose along with doxycycline, 100 mg taken by mouth b.i.d. Another selection for a man who is 17 years of age or older who does not have gonococcal or chlamydial infection will be ofloxacin, 200–400 mg taken by mouth b.i.d. for 10 days OR levofloxacin, 500 mg taken orally q.d. for 10 days.

Men older than 35:

For a man older than 35 years old, use trimethoprim/sulfamethoxazole in one double-strength pill taken by mouth b.i.d. OR ciprofloxacin, 250–500 mg used every day for 10 days. Use medicine for 4 weeks when the man also has prostatitis.

Benign prostatic hyperplasia

Medicine needs to lessen the mass and/or quality of the gland. Medicine includes terazosin, 1 mg taken orally before going to sleep (may be augmented up to 10 mg before going to sleep); prazosin, 1 mg taken orally b.i.d. to t.i.d. (augmented up to 6–15 mg daily); doxazosin, 1 mg taken each day (go to 16 mg when needed); finasteride, 5 mg taken by orally every day; tamsulosin, 0.4 mg taken orally every day. The patient may have balloon enlargement of the urethra in the prostate.

Fibrocystic breast changes

Use warm pads, eat less salt, and utilize diuretics before menstruation. Utilize vitamin E in amounts of 400–600 mg international units taken orally every day, vitamin B_6, 50–100 mg every day. Use evening primrose oil, 100 mg every day. The use of hormonal and antihormonal treatment is debatable, but if the condition is significant, the choices are: contraceptives taken orally with small amount of estrogen and comparatively large amount of progesterone, danazol, bromocriptine, and tamoxifen. Surgery is an option, but this is often debatable.

Breast cancer

The patient needs to see an oncologist. The medical treatment is contingent upon how far the tumor has progressed, existence of hormone receptors, and the indications that the woman is experiencing along with what she would rather do. Medical attention can be in the form of an operation, chemotherapy, radiation treatment, and/or hormone treatment.

Dysfunctional uterine bleeding

Depends upon severity of condition and the age of the patient. The patient may need to see a doctor. To stop heavy and significant or ongoing bleeding, the patient may need an IV of conjugated estrogens and then combined birth control taken orally or medroxyprogesterone acetate to stop it from happening again. Inducing ovulation is only used for someone that wants to get pregnant, in which case clomiphene citrate is utilized. Use iron supplements when necessary. The patient needs to keep a record of basal body temperature and make an account of indications when the problem arises.

Dysmenorrhea

A primary case will need: prostaglandin synthetase inhibitors (PGSI), birth control taken orally (if the patient is having intercourse), medium amount of habitual physical activity, nutrition that has a lot of whole grains, beans, vegetables and fruits, and cutting out salt, sugar, and caffeine from the diet. Other choices include omega-3 fatty acids, thiamine (B_1), magnesium supplements, and vitamin E. Secondary case will need treatment depending on what is causing the condition.

Endometriosis

Utilize combined small amount of estrogen monophasic oral birth control used on an ongoing basis so that the menstrual period will stop, nonsteroidal anti-inflammatory drugs to aid the pain. Medroxyprogesterone acetate (MPA) in an amount of 30 mg taken orally every day will make the endometrial tissue waste away, depot MPA used 100–400 mg intramuscularly each month makes endometrial tissue waste away. Danazol, 200–400 mg taken orally twice a day causes the absence of ovulation and makes the menstrual periods stop, and GnRH-agonists may be used for the same reason. Operation options include removal of endometrial implants with laser or electrocautery and hysterectomy utilizing salpingo-oophorectomy (which restores the woman to health in 90% of cases).

Pap smear results

If results fall inside regular limits, do the test again every year or when needed as determined by danger elements and patient age. The majority of cellular alterations are due to inflammation. Other causes could include deterioration and flare-up associated with atrophic vaginitis, the utilization of an IUD, radiation, or diethylstilbestrol exposure in utero.

- If there is infection, manage it depending on what is creating the problem and do the test again in a year.
- If there are reactive or reparative alterations, then manage any infection and know that it might be linked to a birth control device like an IUD, deterioration alterations, chemotherapy and/or radiotherapy or other, and the patient will need another Pap in 4–6 months.
- If there is low- and high-grade SIL, do colposcopy and cervical biopsies including ECC, check mild lesions using Pap assessments twice a year for 2 years (as long as the ECC is negative), and the regular management may be cryotherapy, large loop excision or transformation zone (LLETZ), or laser vaporization. This patient might need to see a doctor if carcinoma in situ may be present.
- If there are atypical squamous cells of undetermined significance (ASCUS), there is a 10%–40% chance of getting SIL, and 5%–10% of these cases will be HSIL. Do the Pap test again in 4-6 months (three times in a row), do colposcopy and cervical biopsies including ECC when there is HSIL or if the patient has HIV, and if the patient is perimenopausal or postmenopausal, use vaginal estrogen cream before doing the Pap again or before doing a colposcopy. Do this even when the patient is using HRT. The patient needs to see a doctor if there is squamous cell carcinoma, adenocarcinoma, or another epithelial or nonepithelial malignant neoplasm. For a hormonal assessment, handle any deterioration.

Amenorrhea

The treatment will be contingent upon what is causing the problem, and a consultation with a doctor is frequently needed.

Premenstrual syndrome

Pyridoxine, multivitamins, diuretics when the patient has an issue with too much fluid being kept inside, progesterone (debatable, because some research says that it does not work any better than a placebo), prostaglandin inhibitors, oral birth control, danazol, bromocriptine (used for breast pain), and selective serotonin reuptake inhibitors (SSRIs) if the patient has a significant condition.

Peptic ulcer disease

In order to get rid of *Helicobacter pylori*, use antimicrobials. For pain, use proton pump inhibitors, because they help the pain faster and give quicker remedy than an H_2 receptor antagonist. H_2 receptor antagonists are utilized. Use antacids mainly to go along with antisecretory medications. Use anticholinergics in very uncommon cases under a doctor's care to help refractory pain. Use sucralfate (mucosal protectant). Medical attention of antacids, H_2 receptor antagonists, or sucralfate gives an outcome of a total remedy for 90%–95% of patients after 2–3 months.

Gastroesophageal reflux disease

Phase I – Antacids (which are used instead of proton pump inhibitors for the majority). Use 80–100 mEq of neutralizing activity following eating and prior to sleep. Antacid liquid is favored over tablets.

Phase II – When regular medication does not work, use proton pump inhibitor. Although H$_2$ antagonists do not work as well, they may be utilized just as with peptic ulcer disease.

Phase III – When phase II medications are not enough, see a doctor about more assessments and utilize stronger medical attention such as an increased dose of the proton pump inhibitor, prokinetic for heightening the LES tone, esophageal motility, and gastric emptying.

Phase IV – Operation may be needed if the patient has stricture, bleeding, pulmonary aspiration, or significant refractory indications.

Prokinetics:
Gastroesophageal reflux disease – Prokinetics heighten LES tone, esophageal motility, and gastric emptying. Medications for this are:
- Metoclopramide, 10–15 mg prior to eating and sleeping, but these have a lot of adverse outcomes such as tiredness, fretfulness, bewilderment and extrapyramidal responses.
- Cisapride, 10 mg prior to eating or sleeping, acts synergistically along with H$_2$ receptor antagonists to help mending. Death-inducing cardiovascular issues can happen if used along with medication that inhibits cytochrome P450 3A4 enzymes and/or if comorbidities make the patient more likely to have dysrhythmias.
- Bethanechol, 25 mg, half an hour prior to eating, but it only works in a restricted way and should not be used at all if the patient has asthma, ischemic heart disease, or urinary retention.

Diverticulitis

Use broad-spectrum antibiotics including anaerobic activity for 7–10 days or pending the time when the indications improve. These may be amoxicillin/clavulanate potassium, 875 mg/125 mg b.i.d. Another choice is metronidazole, 500 mg t.i.d. plus ciprofloxacin, 500 mg b.i.d. or trimethoprim-sulfamethoxazole, 160/180 mg b.i.d. The patient should rest in bed while there are indications of this condition. See a doctor about going to the hospital if the condition does not begin to improve within 72 hours, the body temperature is over 102°, there are other assessments necessary, or the patient is elderly. If the condition is significant and the patient needs to go to the hospital, use antibiotics, rest the bowels, and get an IV to hydrate the body.

Psychoactive substance abuse

Generally none. Otherwise, haloperidol for psychotic or violent patients. Diazepam may lessen muscle tremors or agitation. Phenothiazine neuroleptics should NOT be used for patients who have used PCP. Vitamin C or cranberry juice can help make urine more acidic and help get PCP out of the body.

Viral hepatitis

- A case with no complexities needs mostly accommodating measures, rather than medication.
- Antiemetics – Use half an hour prior to eating to help queasiness and vomiting; rectal might be handled better than oral medication.
- Vitamin K – For someone with raised PT.
- HCV – Use combination treatment including pegylated interferon and ribavirin; medical attention is complicated and protocol alters often, so see an expert for latest counsel. The way it works is not known. This can eliminate the virus for up to 5/10 patients if it is genotype 1 or up to 8/10 patients if it is genotype 2 or 3. It works better in patients with low serum titer HCV RNA, in patients who are not elderly, in females, or patients with a lack of cirrhosis. There is no information about survival rates or stopping the worsening to ongoing active hepatitis.

Acute gastroenteritis

Generally antiemetics or antidiarrheal medications are not needed and could actually make the condition last longer. Medicating someone with salmonella could make the carrier condition last longer. Use IV medication when required. See a doctor if symptoms do not improve after 2 days. Look for stool ova and parasites. You may have to do particular stool cultures and proctosigmoidoscopy. Make an account of bacterial infections or food poisoning to the health department. Antibiotics are not encouraged, but may be needed if the condition goes on for 3 or 4 days, the patient is having 8–10 bowel movements every day, or if there is an irregular immune reaction.

Irritable bowel syndrome

Talk to a doctor prior to barium enema or proctosigmoidoscopy. Medications include:
- Bulk laxatives.
- Anticholinergics.
- Loperamide or another opiate –for very acute conditions; likelihood for patients to misuse this medication is high.
- Tricyclic antidepressants.
- 5-HT_3 antagonists.

Colorectal cancer

The patient will need any tumors removed with an operation or a resection, the choice of which is contingent upon how deep is the cancer is. If it has spread when the problem is identified, there is a more negative prediction for the future, and palliative medical attention will be needed. If the patient needs resection, there is commonly a need for temporary colostomy. Watch the patient for indications of not enough body fluid while getting colon preps.

Colon cancer screening:

The American Cancer Society advises colon cancer screens for patients with an average chance of getting it, starting when the patient turns 50. This includes assessments for fecal mysterious blood every year, flexible sigmoidoscopy done in 5-year increments, double-contrast barium enema done in 5-year increments, and colonoscopy done in 10-year increments.

Medication with elderly patients

An elderly patient has more of a chance of adverse effects. Approximately 1/3 hospitalizations that are related to side effects of drugs and 1/2 drug-associated fatality happen in patients that at least 60 years of age. In the United States, expenses for prescriptions for elderly patients make up 30% of every prescription filled and 40%–50% for non-prescription drugs. Elderly patients spend more than $3 billion annually on these medications. Most have at least one ongoing problem, including arthritis, high blood pressure, heart problems, diabetes, or other conditions. Many need more than one drug for treatment. There are more adverse drug reactions (ADR), and 30% of elderly patients who are not in the hospital have these side effects, 10% of whom will need to go to the hospital for treatment for the side effects. Frequently seen adverse reactions include edema, queasiness, vomiting, anorexia, vertigo, loose stools, infrequent and difficult stools, bewilderment, and urinary retention. Be careful not to misidentify these as another condition or symptom of aging.

Physiological alterations:

There is less albumin concentration. Because drugs commonly bind to protein (rather than fat), this is significant. Less albumin reduces the amount of places that can bind to protein and makes more free drug in plasma. This can cause an elderly patient to get too much of a drug. Problems include less tolerance for normal amounts of medication including toxicity arising even with less of the medication used, lowered metabolism (generally liver since it is smaller and does not have as much blood flow), less absorption due to lessened liver enzyme work and time it takes for gastric area to empty as well as higher gastric pH, a range of distribution, and lessened capability for getting the medication out of the system due to decreased glomerular filtration rate (GFR). The GFR decreases by half somewhere between the ages of 30 and 90.

Issues with medication:
- Reason for it.
- Medication is dependable.
- Smallest time.
- Smallest dose.
- Affordable.
- Makes the patient's life better.
- Stay away from side effects.
- Assess if using correctly.
- Find someone else to help when needed.
- Utilize organizers, book of days, and/or big font.
- Use tools to help giving the medications (like a spacer for an inhaler).

Difficulties with medication:
- Overuse of prescription medications.
- Medication adherence and compliant issues (e.g., providing incorrect or incomplete past medical history to the professional, or using medicine that is out of date, changing dose without doctor's orders to do so).
- Misunderstanding of how the medicine is supposed to be used due to problems understanding, not being able to hear the direction, or receiving insufficient information.
- Not remembering the reason, amount, or how often the drug should be used. This may result in repeating the medicine when it has already been taken.
- Cost.
- Vision issues can result in misreading the label and taking wrong dosage.

- Problems getting the bottle open, dealing with small pills, cutting pills in half, and using inhalers.
- More than one medical worker or more than one pharmacy can lead to inadvertent redundancy of the same medication, as can using the generic and brand name of the same thing at the same time.

<u>Histamine blockers:</u>

Adverse effects include paradoxical central nervous system provocation that has an outcome of ataxia in elderly patients.

<u>Antihistamines:</u>

May cause problems with sight and walking, causing a fall, as well as fuzzy mental ability and an influence on ability to function, which may cause unforeseen hospital visits or having to go to a nursing home. Also can interfere with other medications or make other medications have worse side effects.

Adverse outcomes of prescription medications

Bewilderment	digoxin, cimetidine, dopamine agent, antihistamine, hypnotic, sedative, anticholinergic, anticonvulsant
Anorexia	digoxin
Low energy or weakness	diuretic, antidepressant, antihypertensive
Absentmindedness	barbiturate
Difficult bowel movements	anticholinergic
Loose stool	oral antacid

GI upset	iron, NSAID, salicylate, corticosteroid, estrogen, alcohol
Ringing in the ears (tinnitus)	analgesic
Urinary retention	anticholinergic, alpha-agonist
Orthostatic low blood pressure	antihypertensive, sedative, diuretic, antidepressant
Depression	benzodiazepine
Vertigo	sedative, antihypertensive, anticonvulsant, diuretic

Antidepressants

Tertiary Tricyclic Antidepressants:
- Amitriptyline
- Clomipramine
- Doxepin
- Imipramine
- Trimipramine

Secondary Tricyclic Antidepressants:
- Amoxapine
- Desipramine
- Nortriptyline
- Protriptyline

SSRIs:
- Fluoxetine
- Fluvoxamine
- Sertraline
- Paroxetine

MAO:
- Phenelzine
- Tranylcypromine

Other:
- Alprazolam
- Bupropion
- Nefazodone
- Trazodone
- Venlafaxine

Antianxiety drugs

The average daily dose is split into 2–4 parts during the day. Elderly patients need smaller amounts. Medication-resistant patients could need a lot more than the amounts listed below. These amounts are the averages.

Benzodiazepines: Work longer:
- Chlordiazepoxide – 15–40 mg
- Clorazepate dipotassium – 15–60 mg
- Diazepam – 4–40 mg
- Halazepam – 60–160 mg

Benzodiazepines: Shorter acting, used for the elderly or with lessened clearance):

- Alprazolam – 0.75–1.5 mg
- Lorazepam – 2–6 mg
- Oxazepam – 30–60 mg

Nonbenzodiazepine:
- Buspirone – 20–30 mg
- Hydroxyzine – 30–300 mg
- Meprobamate – 400–2000 mg
- Paroxetine – 40 mg

To treat aggression and mania:
- Carbamazepine – Begin with 100–200 mg, then up titrate to 400–1500 mg pending the serum level reaching 8–12 ug/mL.

Delirium

There is no particular medication that works optimally. You may use sensible amount of a sedative to help the patient sleep, lessen stress, and lessen disturbance or fidgetiness. Short-acting anxiolytics with no active metabolites may be used, including:
- Oxazepam, 10–50 mg daily
- Lorazepam, 0.5–2 mg daily
- Alprazolam, 0.5–4 mg daily

To quickly compose the patient that is very disturbed, use haloperidol, 0.5 mg in an IV together with 0.5–1 mg of lorazepam. Repeat after half an hour and continue until the patient becomes composed. When the delirium cycle stops, you can continue the use of sedatives on the patient, especially for evening and night.

Bursitis

When the result of an injury, use a splint, heat for half an hour t.i.d. or q.i.d., and use ASA or NSAID (Naproxen, 250 mg b.i.d. or t.i.d.). When the problem comes back and fluid gathers again, inject long acting corticosteroids. When the condition is caused by infection, cut, drain, and use parenteral antibiotics.

Osteoarthritis

Use acetaminophen, 500 mg–1 g t.i.d. or q.i.d.; nonsteroidal anti-inflammatory drugs (NSAIDs) such as ibuprofen, 400–800 mg t.i.d., indomethacin, 50–200 mg daily to a maximum of 1 g q.i.d. Think about using an H_2 blocker if the patient is utilizing NSAID. Adverse outcomes of NSAID are gastrointestinal problems, retaining water, platelet irregularities, or hepatic and renal abnormality. An operation may be needed, in which case a doctor should be seen regarding surgical methods like fusion or joint replacement.

Rheumatoid Arthritis

Disease-modifying antirheumatic drugs (DMARDS), for which methotrexate is favored with a supplement of Folate, 1 mg every day or 7 mg once a week; antimalarials (such as hydroxychloroquine sulfate); gold salts (either in the muscle or taken orally); corticosteroids, in amounts not higher than 10 mg of prednisone or something similar daily for a temporary amount of time to alleviate disabling indications; intra-articular corticosteroids when other drugs are not enough.

Gout

NSAID: indomethacin, 50 mg in 8-hour increments pending improvement of symptoms; Colchicine helps the most in the initial 24–48 hours, use 0.5–0.6 mg taken orally each hour pending improvement of pain, development of GI indications, or reaching the maximum dose of 6 mg; corticosteroids are utilized if the patient is unable to use an NSAID; analgesics like codeine or meperidine might be needed, but do NOT use ASA. The patient should rest in bed for 24 hours after the time that an acute attack goes away. Use nutrition to keep up an every-day elimination of 2000 cc of urine. Avoid obesity and dehydration. A low purine nutritional plan does not influence blood levels much at all. The patient will need support to keep up the medical plan. Continue with good nutrition. Preventative drugs include uricosuric medication: probenecid, 0.5 g daily, slowly using more to 1–2 g daily (stay away from utilizing with salicylates); allopurinol, 100 mg daily used for 7 days in the beginning, then 200–300 mg every day (watch out for rash).

Osteoporosis

Estrogen for prevention. Another medication may be used with estrogen to handle vasomotor indications or vulva/vaginal deterioration. These should be temporary (5 years). Progestin is necessary if the female has an intact uterus. Use bisphosphonates to stop osteoclast mediated bone resorption, for prevention and for the condition: alendronate and risedronate are used a minimum of 30 minutes before ingesting food with 8 oz of water. Salmon calcitonin lessens bone resorption but is used only for medical attention (not prevention) to relieve bone pain problems. Selective estrogen receptor modulators (SERMS) are both preventative and used to handle the condition as an agonist and antagonist for estrogen receptors (Raloxifene). SERMS have an estrogen type of influence on bone and lipid levels, but estrogen antagonist influence for breast and endometrial tissue. Calcium is needed for both sexes in amounts of: 1300 mg daily for ages 13–18; 1000 mg daily for ages 19–50; 1000–1500 mg daily. Take 400-600 IU of vitamin D every day. Ways to get calcium: nutrition, calcium carbonate (least costly), calcium citrate (absorbs well), or calcium phosphate (not as much constipation).

Epicondylitis

(Tennis Elbow) – To alleviate pain, use mild pain medication, relaxation, and ice on the area. Use a counterforce brace or splint on the wrist. Use peritendon cortisone into the area. If the pain keeps on, eliminate all motion to the area for 6–8 weeks by utilizing a cast that has 90° elbow flexion. Use physical therapy for getting the area stronger and to increase movement after the cast comes off. Strengthen with physical activity to train the muscles on the forearm and wrist. When linked to a physical activity, identify whether an inappropriate method of doing the activity is accountable for the harm. When these techniques do not work, an operation may be needed.

Carpal tunnel syndrome

Raise the area, use a splint, and put corticosteroids into the area when bursitis is also an issue. See a doctor if an operation is needed. Talk to the healthcare provider if the condition gets worse. Use NSAID with food and make an account of gastric problems that arise. Think about altering the type of work that caused the problem.

Knee pain

Take it easy, use cold, and keep the knee from moving. Use NSAID medication. Range of movement (ROM) on the knee should be done to keep the area from getting rigid. Medical attention includes quadriceps setting, aspirate effusion, and checking the ROM and doing activities to make the muscles stronger. When ACL/PCL tears do not get better, see an orthopedic surgeon.

Ankle sprain

The medical attention is contingent upon how bad the harm is. The main thing needed is taking it easy, icing the area for 15-20 minutes in increments of 1-2 hours apart for 72 hours, and then starting contrast baths. Put pressure on it and raise it. Do not put weight on it. Use NSAID for 10-14 days. Start ROM if there are no indications. If it is grade 1 or 2, look at it again in 7-10 days. If it is grade 3, a cast is needed. Begin rehabilitation the day following the harm, on a patient-to-patient basis. Rehabilitation includes ROM, Achilles tendon stretches, isometric exercises, manual resistance activities and working on the ankle strength.

Low back pain

To alleviate hurting, use salicylates or acetaminophen; nonsteroidal anti-inflammatory drugs (NSAIDs); opiates in some circumstances. Medicine used to loosen up the muscles may be used temporarily (1–2 weeks), but stay away from these if the patient is older. For radiculopathy, the initial medication is 5-day steroid dose pack. Make an appointment for another check-up a week later. When the patient has not gotten better in that week, he should see an expert to get an epidural steroid injection (ESI). Traction is another alternative. Use back and abdominal physical activity to keep it from happening or coming back. Do not do these exercises when an attack is occurring. Walking is more useful for this condition than running. Back rubs can help. Sometimes the patient has a psychosocial issue that adds to the problem, such as anxiety, depression, family aggression, no coping mechanisms, or marriage and family issues. The patient can go back to his or her job as long as action is restricted. They must learn to handle stress.

Muscle strain

Instruct the patient to take it easy on the area and use tools when necessary. Use ice t.i.d. for 20 minutes at a time. Put pressure on the area, raise it, and take pain medication. NSAID medication may be used.

Anemias

Iron deficiency anemia:
Treat the condition creating the problem. Look for bleeding if there is vitamin deficiency or poor nutrition. Consider infection, injury, neoplasm, or GI problems. Consider more assessments when necessary (stool guaiac, bilirubin, or other). See a doctor if Hct is < 25%/dL, positive stool guaiac or prior bleeding, other patients in the family have anemia, condition with flare-up, infection or malignancy, or symptoms do not improve with the use of

iron supplements. Use oral iron pills, and if that is not sufficient or if the patient cannot use it, use parenteral iron (more costly and has worse adverse effects).

Macrocytic anemias:

(MCV > 100 u^3) – Medical attention includes the use of B$_{12}$ (cyanocobalamin), 100 ug IM q.d. for a week, then lessen how often it is used and give a total of 2000 ug in the initial 6 weeks of treatment. After that, the patient will need to use 100 ug IM every month for the rest of the lifespan. Some patients need cobalamin taken by mouth in a large dose (1000 ug daily) to substitute for parenteral in the maintenance phase, but it must be ingested every day without fail. When the anemia is significant, the patient might require K$^+$ supplements to keep from getting low potassium levels. Check back with elderly patients or patients who have cardiovascular indications within in 48 hours following initiation of treatment. Quickly raised RBC creation might cause too much fluid in the blood for patients with these factors. Consider using simultaneous iron supplements in the initial month. Quick blood cell regeneration raises how much iron is needed and can cause a lack of iron in the body.

<u>Folic acid deficiency anemia:</u>

The patient should use folate, 1 mg taken orally or otherwise daily. The length of time to take it is contingent upon what is causing the condition and the time it takes to correct the deficiency. When it is linked to problems with absorption, (like Sprue), use a maximum of 5 mg daily. A large amount of folic acid can fix hematological irregularities when the B$_{12}$ is lacking, but it will not fix neurological problems.

<u>Sickle cell anemia:</u>

See a doctor if the patient may have this condition so that they may get medical attention. Supportive medical attention includes ongoing folic acid supplements, cytotoxic agents to lessen how often incidences occur, and antibiotics for prevention. To handle significant pain incidences, use analgesia, high-volume IV liquids, oxygen for handling hypoxia, antibiotics for handling linked bacterial infections, and blood transfusions when the patient has aplastic or hemolytic problems, or in the last trimester of pregnancy.

Leukemia

See a doctor if there is a chance that a patient has this condition. The objective of treatment will be remission. Utilize chemotherapy and bone marrow transplant. Give the patient help with emotional requirements. Give the patient and their family help with handling ongoing issues with this condition, such as reliance, withdrawal, alteration in who is accountable for things, different ways of looking at one's body, or other issues.

Non-Hodgkin's lymphoma

Medical attention is contingent upon the grade and severity of the condition. The treatment includes radiotherapy, chemotherapy, and bone marrow transplant. More current modalities are monoclonal antibodies (Mabs) by themselves and together with radionuclides or toxins so that cytotoxic effects are created. Cytokines (e.g., interferons), tumor necrosis factor, and interleukin 2 are now under investigation for treatment of this condition. The prediction for the future is generally not as optimistic as Hodgkin's.

Antihistamines

When using this medicine, the patient needs to be told not to take other over-the-counter drugs unless talking to a nurse practitioner or pharmacist first. Some over-the-counter drugs (including herbs) could have a negative reaction with this medication. Make sure you have a complete record of what the patient is already taking before prescribing this medicine. Also, warn the patient about using topical antihistamines for a long time. An antihistamine will not influence circulating histamine, so the patient will need to stay away from any identified allergens. If the patient experiences constipation or urinary retention, they should get in touch with the nurse practitioner. For a child who has allergic rhinitis, a good choice is brompheniramine (Dimetane) or diphenhydramine (Benadryl). Benadryl will make the child sleepier.

Loratadine

Loratadine (Claritin) – Generally prescribed to be taken one time a day, which is a benefit because the patient is more likely to follow through with the regimen. However, it does cost more than some other first-generation antihistamines.

Steroids

Patients using steroids for a long time need to be checked for adrenal shortage in the event of a significant sickness (as this causes more stress). Raise the dose to 60 mg daily, and then gradually pull it back to 10 mg daily. If this problem occurs, use stress-dose corticosteroids for the time that the patient is sick. Quitting the medicine or keeping it equal to the same level that it was could provoke acute adrenal shortage.

Gout

Utilize Colchicine, 0.6 mg q.i.d.

<u>Acute gout:</u>
Use NSAIDs if appropriate for the patient.

Fosamax

Used for calcium absorption, as in a patient with osteoporosis. It may cause gastritis or mouth ulcers, in which case the medication should be discontinued.

Fibromyalgia

Warmth and rub-down, although not on any trigger areas. Medically handle patient indications. Medicine includes amitriptyline (Elavil), NSAIDs, cyclobenzaprine (Flexeril), temazepam (Restoril), and triazolam (Halcion). Easy physical exertion is advised, which is best done in the afternoon or evening in a low-impact form.

Joint injury

Use RICE: Rest, Ice, Compression, and Elevation. Some patients may also need an x-ray, medication for pain, NSAID, physical therapy, or to go and see a specialist for an MRI.

Female rape case

Take time to give the patient information. It is dangerous to make her go face-to-face with the attacker to get medical records. Postexposure prophylaxis (PEP) is a good choice and will work. Rape is traumatic and gives the woman more of a chance of getting a disease, including HIV.

Side effects of medication

A fully grown patient has more chance for side effects, and this is due to using more kinds of medication, being exposed to more, and the natural effects of age on the immune system. Patients with previous bad responses to drugs will have more of a chance of it happening again with another medication. The chance of side effects happens in the initial 2–3 weeks of use.

***Pneumocystis carinii* pneumonia prevention**

Use trimethoprim-sulfamethoxazole (Septra, Bactrim) for both medically handling and preventing this condition. Generally it is used for 21 days. It can be 7–10 days before a reaction to the medication is noticed.

Nasal decongestants

Use for more than 3 days may have a rebound outcome when the patient stops utilizing the medicine. This can cause more congestion due to reflex vasodilation. This might go on for 2–3 weeks before signs of improvement.

Second-generation antihistamines

The main benefit is that these medications cannot go over the blood/brain barrier, so they will not create sleepiness or a problem with psychomotor activity. There is not as much of a problem with dry mouth or constipation, and they give little anticholinergic activity. The disadvantage is that it is 15–30 times more expensive. These drugs are quickly absorbed (1–2 hours after taking orally without food).

Adenosine

The American Heart Association's Advanced Cardiac Life Support (ACLS) advises the use of adenosine as the best alternative for patients in need of immediate medical attention for supraventricular tachycardia as long as the patient has a blood system that is fine and secure. Supraventricular tachycardia is described as quick heart rate that comes from the upper heart chambers and can cause an insufficient amount of blood to get to the body. Use adenosine 6 mg IV push.

Lovastatin

Lovastatin (trade name: Mevacor) is a cholesterol-lowering drug; most effective time of day to take this medication is in the evening, because the majority of cholesterol becomes synthesized during the hours from midnight to 3:00 AM.

Procainamide and hydralazine

Procainamide (Pronestyl) and hydralazine (Apresoline) can create indications that are a lot like lupus. Stopping the use of these will make the indications go away.

Malaria prevention

Use chloroquine phosphate, 5 mg/kg of body weight with a maximum of 300 mg for a fully grown patient.

Allergic rhinitis

Use antihistamines, and instruct the patient to stay away from the allergen to lessen the problem. To get more management and to steady the mast cells, use corticosteroids.

<u>Erythromycin ethylsuccinate and astemizole:</u>
These should NOT be used at the same time and can cause dysrhythmias that may lead to death.

Sympathomimetics

Used for allergic rhinitis to create vasoconstriction and lessen fluid, swelling, and emissions.

Cromolyn sodium

Utilized for getting the mast cell membrane to be stable and to block histamine at the time that the cell is exposed to an antigen.

GERD

This condition is initially treated with weight loss. Also, utilize ranitidine (Zantac), 150 mg b.i.d. Changes in the way one lives is the best way to handle this condition.

PUD

As long as the condition has no complications, start with omeprazole (Prilosec), 20 mg q.d. The aim is to alleviate the symptoms, give a remedy for the ulcer, and not be too expensive.

Shigellosis

Handle by treating the patient indications, and use trimethoprim-sulfamethoxazole (Septra) in amounts appropriate for the patient's age and weight b.i.d. for 7–10 days. The medicine will make the problem go away faster and will stop it from moving to another place. Drink plenty of fluids (because diarrhea may cause dehydration) for 2–4 days, do not have dairy, do have electrolyte-filled sports liquids, and eat as needed. Do not take antidiarrheal drugs, as they may negatively affect intestinal motility.

Mild ulcerative colitis

Utilize sulfasalazine (Azulfidine), which helps the patient indications for 50%–75% of patients. When there is not a reaction after 2–4 weeks, add prednisone.

Giardiasis

As long as it is a fully grown patient who is not pregnant, use boiling water and quinacrine (Atabrine), 100 mg PO t.i.d. for 5 days.

Vomiting

Use Emetrol, 15–30 mL PO for a fully grown patient. For a child (> 12 years old), use Phenergan, 25 mg, but do not give to patients younger than 6 years of age). For an older child or fully grown patient, use hydroxyzine hydrochloride (Vistaril), 25–100 mg. Trimethobenzamide (Tigan) may be sued (200 mg).

Pepto-Bismol

A common side effect is stool that is darker than usual.

Uric acid renal calculus

The diet is very hard to follow, because it is an alkaline-ash, low purine diet. The majority of patients will not eat that way even when they understand that the condition is more likely to come back if they do not. Medication that may be prescribed for it as an alternative includes allopurinol (Zyloprim) 100 mg q.d. PO. Check the serum uric acid amounts to make sure they are staying regular and to manage any uric acid stones. This will let the patient eat more normally.

Oxybutynin

Used for someone that has frequent needs to urinate. Side effects include anticholinergic outcomes, like dry mouth. Other drugs taken at the same time, such as diuretics, can make the effects worse. Eating hard candy or chewing gum can help the dry mouth. If the anticholinergic outcomes are extremely strong due to taking another medicine that also causes anticholinergic outcomes, the patient may have a chance of falling. Go over the other drugs that the patient is taking very meticulously before adding anything else.

Medications causing incontenence

May get incontinence with the use of hypnotics, sedatives, or antidepressants. The first 2 medications cause sedation and muscles that are more relaxed than usual. This is true for everyone, but an older patient can be more affected due to the effects of aging on the central nervous system. There is more muscle relaxation. Antidepressants give anticholinergic outcomes and can cause sedation as well.

Medications causing impotence

Antihypertensive medications, such as propranolol (Inderal, Inderal LA), may cause impotence.

Nitrofurantoin

Nitrofurantoin (Macrodantin) – Should not be used when there is a problem with renal ability, when there is not enough antibacterial concentration in the urine, or when there is more of a chance of toxicity. If a patient has an ongoing UTI, consider using this drug for prevention, 100 mg PO, qhs. If the patient is elderly, have no serum or tissue gathering for this medication.

<u>Adverse outcomes:</u>
Adverse outcomes include gastrointestinal discomfort, but this may be helped by taking with food or milk. Many patients experience an odd color to the urine. Keep using the drug for a minimum of 3 days after getting a sterile urine sample. Make sure the patient knows that this drug can make oral contraception ineffective.

Renal calculi

Handle pain first. Use morphine sulfate, 10 mg SC or meperidine (Demerol). Ibuprofen (Advil) can be used if the pain is just starting. Trimethobenzamide (Tigan) may be utilized after the pain regimen has begun.

Phenazopyridine

(Pyridium) – Used for problems with urination, frequency, and urgency. If the patient notices that the sclera in the eyes starts to change into a shade of yellow, then they need to come back to the clinic right away. The drug can also stain contact lenses yellow. It is a sign of poor renal excretion, and the patient will need a total renal checkup including renal panel, parathyroid hormone (PTH), magnesium, thyroid-provoking hormone, and serum calcium measurements. Get a 24-hour urine collection to check creatinine. The patient might need to see a nephrologist. Take this drug with food.

Oxybutynin

(Ditropan) – Do NOT use if the patient has narrow-angle glaucoma. It may be used if the patient has open-angle glaucoma.

ACE inhibitors

Put more pressure inside the kidneys with renal artery stenosis, so do NOT use this medication if the patient has renal artery stenosis. This medicine is good for shielding a patient who has cardiovascular disease, hypertension, or diabetes.

Balanitis

Use an antifungal medication such as nystatin (Mycostatin) applied to the skin or ciclopirox (Loprox). When needed, use a drug taken orally, such as fluconazole (Diflucan), 150 mg daily or itraconazole (Sporanox), 100 mg daily.

Acute bacterial prostatitis

Use trimethoprim-sulfamethoxazole (TMP-SMX) for a minimum of 30 days to avoid recurrence.

Epididymitis

Use trimethoprim-sulfamethoxazole (TMP-SMX).

Finasteride

(Proscar) – May be given to a man who has a bigger-than-usual prostate and trouble with urinating. It is very important that this medication not be handled by anyone who is pregnant or able to have children. Women who are pregnant should not even deal with crushed tablets, nor should they have contact with sperm from a man that is using this medication.

Peyronie's disease

Start by using vitamin E, 400 IU, b.i.d., because it aids in softening the fibrous tissue. Plaques in this condition are made up of fibrous tissue.

Uncomplicated vulvovaginal candidiasis

You may use fluconazole in one dose, taken orally. It is very convenient to use (more so than a vaginal cream).

Bacterial vaginosis

For someone who is not pregnant, the best alternative is metronidazole vaginal gel.

Menopause

Although there have been some that advise the use of herbs, there have been no controlled studies done regarding the use of herbs for keeping other conditions from arising. Conservative allopathic Western medicine advises HRT to keep the woman from getting osteoporosis. The final decision about whether to use it belongs to the patient, however, so make sure she has all of the information needed to make a good decision for herself. Do weight-bearing physical activities and ingest more calcium. Instruct the patient to stop smoking, as it increases the likelihood of bone loss.

Oral estrogen

May create a hepatic outcome with first-pass metabolism in the liver. A 25% increase in triglycerides is linked to taking estrogen in this manner. Because transdermal estrogen does not have to depend upon gastrointestinal absorption, it does not go through first-pass metabolism. Some patients will do better with the transdermal way of taking the medicine. Be sure to talk to the patient about the pros and cons of taking estrogen.

Birth control methods

IUD:
A very effective method of birth control (more than 99%), and it is easy to use. The patient does not have to have an injection for either putting it in or taking it out. This method is not

advisable for patients who are nulliparous or are not in an ongoing relationship with only one person.

How they work: The way they work is not totally proven, but it has to do with stopping blastocyte implantation by provoking a low-grade endometritis, putting a copper influence on enzymes, making the progesterone work on the endometrium, and keeping the sperm/ovum from moving. A benefit of using a Progesterone T IUD is that the woman will not have as much blood or cramping.

Depo-Provera injections:
Very effective (more than 99%); necessitates an injection in 3-month increments, which may cause the patient not to be as compliant about its use.

Norplant system:
Also more than 99% effective. It necessitates injections to put it in and take it out. Someone with a seizure condition who is taking Phenobarbital or Dilantin should not use this method.

Diaphragm:
88% effective, and necessitates the woman to be actively involved in using it.

Note: this raises the likelihood of getting a UTI and is linked to toxic shock syndrome. Do not use during menstruation, and do not use for more than 24 hours at a time.

Condoms or spermicide:
The only reason that someone should not use either of these is if there is risk of an allergic reaction.

Oral contraception:
Can help shield the woman from ovarian and endometrial cancer. Usually there is not as much bleeding during the woman's period with this method. Some patients have a small amount of

change in weight (3–5 pounds). If the woman has abnormal bleeding, it is commonly fixed by taking a pill that has a stronger or varied progestational agent. A nursing mother should not use combined OCs, because it may lessen the milk that she makes and make it poorer in quality. Nursing mothers can use progestin-only OCs. Women older than 35 and smokers should not take OCs.

How they work: Mainly, they suppress ovulation. This happens for 95%–98% of patients who take them. If ovulation still happens, it can still stop the woman from becoming pregnant by making the cervical mucus thicker which makes the endometrium atrophic, and making the uterus unlikely to accept implantation.

Progestin-only pills: Will not always suppress ovulation, but instead they only suppress it for 40%–60% of cycles. That means they do not work as well as combined contraception pills. They work by making the endometrium atrophy. They can also change the tubal function because of lessening the ovum movement. There is no estrogen in them, so they are a good choice for a nursing mother.

Hormone replacement therapy

Patients with recent diagnosis or occurrence of deep venous thrombosis, ongoing active hepatitis, or irregular genital bleeding for which the cause has not been identified, should not use HRT.

Pelvic inflammatory disease

Use ceftriaxone (Rocephin), 250 mg IM. Use doxycycline (Vibra tabs), 100 mg PO b.i.d. for 10 days. Do CBC and erythrocyte sedimentation rate in order to keep an account of the white blood count and how the body flare-up reaction is going.

Trichomoniasis

Use metronidazole, 2 g PO for one dose. The metronidazole vaginal cream is not sufficient.

Primary dysmenorrhea

Use nonsteroidal anti-inflammatory analgesics. Physical activities, methods of relaxation, heat, and small amounts of oral contraceptives (OCs) may also help.

Gonococcal infection

The majority of cases of PID for females that are engaging in intercourse are gonococcal infections, and they commonly accompany *Chlamydia* infections. Generally you need to medically manage both at the same time. Use ceftriaxone (Rocephin), 125 mg IM and azithromycin (Zithromax), 1 g PO.

Trichomoniasis

The favored method is metronidazole (Flagyl), taken in one 2-g dose. Another choice is using the same dose, but split it into two and to take them both on the same day. The second choice may be better for some patients, as there is not as much nausea, and the patient may be more likely to follow through with it.

Bacterial vaginosis

The favored method is metronidazole (Flagyl), but make sure the patient has not become pregnant. If there is a possibility of pregnancy, do NOT use it.

Health Promotion and Disease Prevention

Hypertension

Life changes:

Advise the patient to lose weight, eat more fruits and vegetables and less fat, eat less than 2.4 g of salt per day, exercise for half an hour every day or the majority of days, limit alcoholic beverages to 2 a day for males or 1 a day for females, and stop smoking.

Coronary artery disease

Risk factors:

Patients have more of a chance of CAD with high blood pressure, smoking, irregular serum lipids, diabetes mellitus, impaired response to insulin and metabolic syndrome, other close relatives with the condition (especially if it begins under age 50), lack of proper exercise, history of taking oral contraceptives, or obesity. The patient's personality may play a role, but this is uncertain. Before 40 years of age, men are more likely to have it (8:1). After the age of 70, men and women are equally at risk (1:1). The total lifespan ratio is 4:1, with men being more likely to get CAD.

Rheumatic fever

Secondary deterrence:

For a reappearing case, some think that getting to the beginning of the second decade of life and having a minimum of 5 years since the patient has had an acute rheumatic fever incident is the time to discontinue prophylactic penicillin except when that patient has a heightened chance of getting a streptococcal infection, such as someone that teaches school or works in a medical profession. Some think that the client needs prophylactic medications for the rest of their life. The best choice for secondary prevention is erythromycin 250 mg PG b.i.d., taken for an indeterminate duration of time.

Pneumonia prevention

- Pneumococcal 23 valent vaccine – Such as pneumovax; 0.5 cc IM – used if the patient is older than 65 years of age or if the patient has an immune problem or an ongoing disease.
- Influenza vaccine – Given every year; can give along with pneumovax on the identical occasion but on dissimilar locations on the body.

Lung cancer prevention

The best way to keep someone from a diagnosis of lung cancer is to prevent it by not smoking. Screening a patient in a routine check-up is not as useful as quitting the use of cigarettes. Today, there is no proof through research and study that screening patients for lung cancer would lessen the death rate due to this condition. The use of bronchoscopy as a way to identify the condition is not a screening test. Rather, it is diagnostic.

Chronic obstructive pulmonary disease

Diet recommendations:
Someone with this condition should eat a high-calorie, high-protein diet with limited, low amounts of carbohydrates. The patient should stay away from carbohydrates as much as possible, because COPD makes the body hang on to carbon dioxide and carbohydrates metabolize into carbon dioxide when they turn into waste.

Patient education

Hyperthyroidism:
The drugs used for this condition will be needed for around 2 years, and they should not be stopped suddenly. When the initial indication of infection or high body temperature arises, discontinue the medication and visit a medical clinic. The drugs used for this condition will

not generally begin to be obvious until the patient has been using them for around 3 weeks. Make sure the patient understands why medications are needed, how much to take, adverse effects, and that the medication may not seem to work for the initial 3 weeks. Give the patient information about diet, including the need to adhere to a high-carbohydrate, high-calorie food plan pending the drugs beginning to work. Stay away from any stimulants (like caffeine). Discuss indications of thyroid storm and hypothyroidism.

Adult hypothyroidism:

Teach the patient about the way the condition works and that it is ongoing. Discuss the fact that medical attention will need to continue throughout the lifespan. Explain why and how medicines are used, including dosing, adverse outcomes, and toxic outcomes. Explain the indications of the condition. Discuss how to handle indications while waiting on the medicine to work. These problems may be how to deal with weariness or dry skin. Discuss the need to eat more fiber and drink more liquid to handle problems with infrequent and difficult stools.

Thyroid nodule:

The information that the patient needs to know will depend on the outcome of the assessments done.

Addison's disease:

Discuss the need to take more cortisol when anxiety is an issue. The patient should keep a card or ID bracelet on their person at all times. Use salt additives when it is very hot or humid. The prediction for the future is great as long as the patient keeps using the medical attention necessary to treat this condition.

Diabetes:

Sick day protocol: Make sure the patient knows that when they are sick, their blood glucose is likely to be higher. This is true even when the patient cannot eat due to being sick. It is necessary to check the blood glucose in 2–4 hour increments. Keep an eye on the urine with regard to ketones when glucose gets to > 240 mg/dL. The patient will need to use more doses or regular insulin on a sick day. Follow the directions for blood glucose levels that are > 240 mg/dL. Do NOT take metformin and acarbose during times of nausea and vomiting. Wait until these symptoms are gone and nutrition is back to normal before taking these medications. Continue checking blood glucose when nausea and vomiting occurs.

Cerebrovascular injury causing loss of control over urination:
Teach the family to institute a planned pattern to help the patient urinate. Getting into a pattern helps to set up management of the problem. Catheters are not the best option because infection may occur. Make sure the patient is still drinking plenty of fluid and do not limit fluids in any way.

Postpolio syndrome:
Instruct the patient to come in for habitual check-ups, and to stay in shape. The patient needs to work out physically until the muscles are sore. They must stay away from cold environments because the cold affects muscle weakness. Aids like canes, walkers, or braces may be utilized. Continue to assess the muscles for strength or weakness.

Syphilis:
Talk to the patient about the regimen that is necessary. Make sure the patient knows that the entire medical plan has to be followed. Do not engage in sex until after the patient and the partner has completed the remedy. Make sure the patient understands how the condition is spread and managed, and advise them to use condoms. Test any syphilis patient for HIV.

Herpes genitalis:
Talk about the medical regimen that is necessary. Encourage the patient not to engage in sex when the condition is occurring. Encourage the use of condoms. Discuss how to keep from getting the condition, how it is spread, and how it is managed. Talk about the risks for pregnancy. Approximately 80% might get viral shedding in times of no indications of this condition.

Genital warts:

Talk about medical and identification routines. Discuss how to avoid it, how it is spread, and how it is medically managed. Advise the patient to keep using condoms. Make sure the patient knows that it is necessary to come back for a check-up, especially if the Pap was irregular. Talk about the likelihood of recurrence, including the fact that the medical management may not work. Discuss recurrence, dormancy, and the lack of indications with viral shedding. Patients who use tobacco experience more difficulty with regard to the recurrence. Smoking and HPV are co elements that link to cervical cancer.

Vulvovaginitis:

Talk about medical attention and identification routines. Do not engage in intercourse pending completion of the medical treatment. Impart information to the patient about how to keep from getting it, how it is acquired, and how it is medically treated. Advise the patient to keep using condoms. Talk about how critical it is to manage BV, trichomoniasis, and any infection when pregnant. Talk about the risks incurred from douching and how often infections occur. Talk about pelvic inflammatory disease (PID) and its link to bacterial vaginosis.

Urinary tract infection:

Talk about medical attention routines and ways to identify the condition. Talk about the need to come back for another check-up when the indications worsen or do not improve with medical attention. Be sure the patient knows that the entire treatment regimen must be finished and that another check-up is needed if the condition comes up again.

Acute pyelonephritis:

Talk about medical attention routines and ways to identify the condition. Discuss the need to finish the whole treatment regimen, and come in for another check-up the next day. The patient needs to drink lots of water. The patient should not engage in sexual intercourse until the entire treatment regimen is finished. Talk about indications that the condition has become significant, what that would look or feel like, and how it is medically handled on an outpatient basis. Discuss the possibility of another instance of this condition arising, which would mean that the patient needs to see the urologist or get a complete assessment.

Acute bacterial prostatitis:

Talk about ways to handle the condition with medicine. Talk about how the condition is identified. Stay away from sex until the problem is managed. Advise the patient to keep using condoms when there is more than one sexual partner. Give information about indications of not being able to void all of the urine and epididymitis. Discuss how essential it is to come back for another check-up.

Epididymitis:

Talk about ways to identify and handle the condition with medicine. Make sure the patient knows that the entire treatment regimen is needed. Encourage the patient not to engage in sexual intercourse until all of the antibiotics are finished. Talk about the puffiness and distress that might go on for weeks or months following getting rid of the cause of infection. Epididymis might stay bigger than normal or stay hardened for an undetermined amount of time. Talk about how to keep from having this condition, how it is spread, and how to handle STDs if that is part of the condition. Advise condoms. Ask the patient about any anxiety or issues.

Benign prostatic hyperplasia:

Talk about ways to identify and handle the condition with medicine. Talk about the indications of urinary retention, kidney failure, and epididymitis. Make sure the patient knows that further check-ups are needed. Stay away from caffeine and alcoholic beverages so that the bladder will not be as aggravated. Stay away from decongestants, antihistamines, tricyclic antidepressants, and anticholinergics.

Prostate cancer:

Make sure the patient gets help as needed for bodily, mental, community, ethnic, situational, and religious issues. Make sure the patient knows that more check-ups are necessary.

Fibrocystic breast changes:

Comfort the patient with the fact that there is only a small chance of malignancy. Talk about how to identify the condition and how it is medically handled. Educate the patient on how to do a breast self-exam, advise her to seek assistance if there is a new accumulation that will not go away after having her period. During check-ups, check for any worsening of the problem and/or simultaneous growth.

Breast cancer:

Talk about ways to identify and handle the condition with medicine. Support the patient in talking about anxiety regarding the condition. Instruct and show her how to do a breast self-exam, and share this information with other relatives, particularly daughters. Advise the patient to get assistance if a new lump is found or if the breast alters. Get the patient help as needed with regard to bodily, mental, sexual, community, ethnic, situational, and religious issues. Make sure the patient understands that further check-ups will be needed.

Dysfunctional uterine bleeding:

Educate the patient about how to check the basal body temperature for record keeping. Talk about treatment and identification of the condition. Talk about how to handle significant or excessive amounts of blood. Go over nutrition needs, including the need to eat a diet that includes more iron. Talk about any worries that the patient may have, and make sure the woman continues to come in for check-ups.

Premenstrual syndrome:

Educate the patient about PMS support groups that are available.

Peptic ulcer disease:

Talk about medical treatment and identification procedures and frequent problems related to treatment. Discuss the reasons for using medications, how much to take, and adverse effects. As far as nutrition, there is no proof that eating bland food or eating small meals more often is needed. Advise the cessation of gastric acid provokers like coffee, soda, or liquids that have caffeine. Stay away from any food or liquid that provokes the problem. Stay away from ingesting food within 3 hours of going to bed so that nighttime provocation of acid can be avoided. Lower anxiety. Discuss the necessity of coming back in if the medicine is not working, there is bleeding, decreased body weight, more weakness, vertigo, or an increase in pain. The use of cigarettes will slow healing. The patient needs to have another check-up in 2–4 weeks to make sure the drugs are working, check for bleeding, and discuss adverse effects of drugs.

Dysplasia and irregular Pap smear:

Talk about medical treatment and identification procedures and frequent problems related to treatment. Advise the patient to get regular Pap smears. Discuss the patient's particular chances of having a problem when appropriate. Instruct the patient about treatment plans and how to handle the condition. Allow the patient to talk about any anxiety.

Gastroesophageal reflux disease:

Talk about how to handle the indications and the aims of treatment. Talk about provoking elements. It will help to lose weight, not eat a lot in one sitting, not do physical activity right after eating, and raise the head when sleeping. Limit alcohol, mint, and orange juice as these slow down the gastric emptying. Limit tomatoes and anything spicy because these can make the patient have heartburn. Try not to bend over after eating. The amount of liquid taken with food has no affect on this condition. Stay away from eating things that are acidic or fatty, like chocolate, peppermint, etc. Make sure the patient has no mistaken beliefs about the reasons for the condition. Instruct the patient about how to use the medication correctly and what adverse outcomes may occur.

Cholecystitis:

Instruct the patient about the condition, what to look forward to, and how it is medically handled. Talk about alterations in indications for which the patient will need to get in touch with a medical expert. These include different types of pain or pain that comes with high body temperature and shivers. Talk about how to use drugs, what they are for, and what adverse outcomes might occur. Discuss diet. When fatty foods come before indications, the patient might need to try eating less fat. Some data indicate that more fiber decreases the risk of developing gallstones. When a patient is in the obese weight range, they should eat to lose weight, but do not try to lose weight quickly, because trendy diets can in reality give more of a chance of developing gallstones, and can provoke significant indications. Advise habitual physical activity because a lack of exercise has been linked to the development of gallstones as well as obesity. Encourage the patient to come back every year for check-ups, and come in when there is a significant attack. Complexities of this condition include empyema, gangrene, and perforation.

Diverticulitis:

Talk about causes, what to anticipate, and medical treatment. Talk about nutrition, including the need to eat a lot of fiber after an acute case. Talk about how eating a lot of fiber could create a problem with bloating and gas in the initial 2 weeks, but that this problem will improve after that time with this type of diet. Stay away from laxatives, enemas, antidiarrheals, or raw, high-residue nutrition. Use bulk-creating elements and stool softeners to keep the condition from coming back. Come back for a check-up in 2–4 days to make sure the problem is getting better with the chosen treatment. Come again after finishing the antibiotic.

Viral hepatitis:

Talk about what to anticipate, how medications are used, and adverse effects. Discuss vitamins that can be used in conjunction with the medications during the condition. Talk about utilizing good hygiene, washing the hands correctly, and getting rid of bodily wastes. Tell the patient not to give blood. Other patients who have been in close contact with the patient need to be assessed. These patients can get immune serum globulin for passive immunity. This immunity will not help after the condition becomes apparent. Come back once a week for two or three weeks, then come back once a month after that when the indications are getting better and the liver is getting better. If the patient is over 40 years of age, more check-ups will be necessary. Complexities in the patient's condition may arise.

Colorectal cancer:

Talk about the chance of colostomy. Support the patient and the family in talking about how they are handling the identification of this condition. Educate the family on places to go for help, such as the American Cancer Society or Ostomy Association.

Depression:

Talk about what to anticipate, how to use medications, and follow-up appointments. The favored method is for the patient to see a mental health expert to get the drugs adjusted and to get at least some psychotherapeutic help. Watch this patient for indications of suicide, shakiness, fuzzy sight, dry mouth, tachycardia, and postural hypotension.

Anxiety:

Talk about what to anticipate and the prediction for the future. Comfort the patient by telling them that this condition does not generally worsen to become something more significant and that medical attention/therapy does help. Anxiety is transitory and can be treated. Talk about how to use the medication. Begin making an account of attacks, including day, time, circumstance, and how bad the indications were (scale of 0–10).

Osteoarthritis:

Talk about how the body works and how to make the muscles stronger. Talk about range of motion movements and ways to lose weight.

Rheumatoid arthritis:

Talk about the autoimmune condition, how to handle stress and unwind, and staying away from alcohol if utilizing methotrexate. Methotrexate should not be used in a pregnant woman or anyone with impaired renal ability. Physical therapy and occupational therapy are helpful. Discuss the ways to handle the condition in regular life.

Gout:

Use ice or heat to aid with symptoms, and raise the influenced region when a significant attack is occurring.

Osteoporosis:

Shield an elderly patient from falling down and make sure the surroundings are not dangerous. Utilize glucocorticoids carefully. Get habitual mammograms and pelvic exams if it is a female using HRT. Talk to youth and young females about getting sufficient amounts of calcium and problems with exercising too much. Handle significant back pain with rest, pain relief, outside support, heating pads, or stool softeners. Stay away from smoking and alcohol.

Bursitis:

Use ice in the initial day. When the inflammation gets better, use wet heat a few times each day.

Muscle strain:

Talk about how to keep the problem from happening again, make sure the patient understands about repetitive motion, and find things that can be altered that would lessen the pressure on the area. Discuss stretching before doing exercise, whether work or athletics.

Iron deficiency anemia:

Talk about reason for problem, how to use medication, side effects, using orange juice or another vitamin C to help absorption, and staying away from milk and antacids as they can inhibit absorption of iron. Eating and drinking with iron supplement could hinder absorption but it might be needed to avoid nausea or upset stomach. Talk about medications bought without a prescription that may cause heart failure or overdose of iron (particularly for incontinence in elderly). Talk about diet and physical activity. The patient will need as much relaxation time as necessary.

Thalassemia:

Talk about indications of too much iron, which include: lethargy, tiredness, lessened amount of body hair, lessened body weight, red palms, bigger male breast tissue, lessened sex drive, stomach pain, skin that is thinner and darker in color, pain or rigidity of joints, fuzzy sight, or another indication associated with the beginning of diabetes, difficulty breathing, or enlarged ankles. The patient should not be subjected to superfluous, repetitive medical tests. The patient should NOT take extra iron.

Leukemia:

Talk about how vital it is to follow directions regarding chemotherapy treatment, what adverse reactions may occur, and how to handle them. Talk about what to anticipate and why the treatment regimen was chosen. Discuss changes due to bodily restrictions.

Anemia of chronic disease:

Talk about the primary reason for this condition and how it links to anemia. Check-ups will depend upon the primary cause. The use of erythropoietin alfa intraveneous or subcutaneous is only for someone that is dependent upon transfusions or someone who would have a much better life because of the outcome.

Macrocytic anemias:

Explain the cause of the condition and what to anticipate. Talk about the requirement of injecting B_{12} for the rest of the lifespan. Give the patient data regarding adverse effects of these injections including pain and fiery feelings on the area of injection, peripheral vascular thrombosis, and temporary loose stools. Talk about CNS indications being reversible when the patient has had them for less than 6 months before starting medical attention. Educate the patient or close relative regarding doing injections or send them to an outpatient facility. Talk about consoling and protection issues if there is also a neurological issue (which may be stopped but cannot be turned back with medical attention). Have a check-up in 4–6 weeks to monitor for hematological reaction. After that, check back in 6 months and do Hct and stool assessments (for occult blood). Do endoscopies in 5-year increments. The chance of getting gastric cancer is greater if the patient has harmful anemia.

Folic acid deficiency anemia:

Talk about the cause and what to expect, necessity of and reason for medical attention, and nutrition that will give the patient folic acid. These food items include asparagus, bananas, fish, green leafy vegetables, peanut butter, beef liver, and wheat bran. Advise the patient to eat these every day, and let them know that cooking these items too long can take away the folic acid. Give the patient a list of these foods. The patient will have to have habitual times of inactivity until the problem is fixed. Talk about properly cleaning the mouth. Follow up with the patient and look at hematological reaction including Hct and reticulocyte amounts in 4–6 weeks. The Hct should start to increase after 2 weeks. The problem should be fixed within 2 months. Patients who do well may get 6–12- month check-ups when the patient has to keep using medical attention.

Delirium:

Support and comfort the patient, and discuss ways to stay out of danger. Reorient the patient. Talk to the patient and relatives about the problem while being comforting and sensitive. Stay away from polypharmacy. Watch how medicine is used and be aware of adverse effects. Encourage the patient to drink enough, make sure there is enough oxygen, and make sure there is a good diet. Evaluate the need for pain management. Manage the atmosphere for stimuli (too much or too little).

Follow-up

Gastric ulcer:

If there was a gastric ulcer, make an account of the remedy of upper GI barium radiograph or endoscopy in 6 weeks if it was a small ulcer and in 12 weeks if it was larger. This is necessary for gastric cases, but not needed for duodenal cases that had no complexities.

Elderly population

In the United States, this word has come to mean anyone at least 65 years of age. From 65–74 years of age is considered young-old; 75–84 is considered middle-old; and 85 years of age or older is considered oldest-old. Elderly female to male ratio (from 2001) is 20.8 million to 14.8 million. Data from 2001 shows that someone who gets to be 65 years old has an anticipated lifespan of 84 years for females or 81 years for males. Males do have higher death rates for each year that they live.

<u>High populations of elderly patients:</u>

Data from 2002 showed that more than 50% of older patients who were not living in institutions did share a home with a husband or wife. The chance of living by oneself or in a residential home increases as the patient gets older. Just 9% of patients who were not in institutions between the ages of 65 and 69 years had to have assistance to do regular daily activities, but 50% of patients from 85 years of age and older needed this type of help. Not many patients in the 65 and older age group went to nursing facilities in 2000, but the number goes up drastically as this population ages, as follows: 1.1% for age 65–74 years, and 18.2% for people age 85 years an older. Data from 2000 showed that nearly 400,000 grandparents older than 65 had the primary care of their grandchildren in their homes. Most patients over 65 years of age reside in cities. Data from 2002 showed that approximately 52% of patients over 65 years of age lived in these states: California, Florida, New York, Pennsylvania, Texas, Ohio, Illinois, Michigan, and New Jersey.

Theories of aging

Aging happens to a patient as time goes by and ends in the patient dying. Some theories regarding aging include: genetic theories, error-catastrophe, DNA, and Hayflick limit or cell aging. Damage theories exist with regard to chemical responses, cross-linkage, and free-radicals. Eventual imbalance theories are about autoimmunity, eventual imbalance and neuroendocrine regulatory system. Other theories involve wear and tear, society, and developmental ideas.

Prevention for the elderly

Although life spans are longer, ongoing diseases are still the primary reason patients die. Elderly patients have more of an absolute chance of getting a disease. They react well to prevention. Keep good records of the patient history, including updating every year and following advice for patients over the age of 65 years. Evaluate nutrition, functional ability, alcoholic beverage intake (more than 2 alcoholic beverages a day constitutes abuse), smoking, illegal drugs, misuse of prescriptions, and exercise level. Preventative measures include a physical, screening assessments, and immunizations. Some routine screenings include: fasting glucose, papanicolaou smear, dipstick urinalysis, mammography, PPD, fecal occult blood/sigmoidoscopy, electrocardiogram, thyroid function, glaucoma and sight, hearing, and cholesterol. Immunizations include yearly flu shot, pneumococcal vaccine, and tetanus. The following screens are controversial: depression for someone with no symptoms, dementia for someone with no symptoms, osteoporosis including bone densitometry for postmenopausal females (counsel females regarding hormone prophylaxis), colon and prostate cancer, and cholesterol for someone with no symptoms.

Work-associated health problems

The most frequently seen type of work-associated health problem is lung disease. Others are repetitive motion injury, hearing loss, cancer, and musculoskeletal harm.

Sports screenings

The only identified gain from this type of screening is to find out if the patient has a risk of an orthopedic injury because of a prior injury.

American Dietetic Association

Nutrition plan:

Bread, cereal, rice, pasta – 6–11 servings; Fruit – 2–4 servings; Vegetable – 3–5 servings; Meat, poultry, fish, dry beans, eggs, nuts – 2–3 servings; Fats, oils, sweets – sparingly.

Immunizations

For healthy, young adults the following immunizations are encouraged:
- Influenza
- Hepatitis B
- Rubella
- Measles
- Tetanus

Prevention for osteoporosis

Prevention methods include good nutrition with no more than 20% protein in the daily plan, more calcium, and less fat. Physical activity should include weight exercises for a minimum of half-an-hour, 3–4 times each week, daily life alterations to allow for more physical activity, and strength activities like swimming or weight machines. Patients should do a moderate amount of walking if there has been osteoporosis identified (contingent upon severity of the condition). Use active or passive range of motion if the patient cannot get out of bed. Estrogen may be used during postmenopausal or post oophorectomy times to lessen the amount of bone resorption.

High-level wellness

A continuum that shows the vibrant interface of health and surroundings at the time that a patient is going in the direction of high-level wellness. The health is vibrant, but there is an ongoing necessity of doing actions that maintain and improve the health.

Maslow's hierarchy of needs

(Maslow, 1954):
- Survival – Food, water, sleep.
- Safety and security – Shield from danger.
- Love and belonging – Affection, camaraderie.
- Self-esteem – Sense of worth, appreciation.
- Self-actualization – Accomplishment of individual potential.

Health belief model

(Becker, 1972) – Health has to do with how old the patient is, gender, race, ethnicity, and salary level. Dangers to health include perceived susceptibility and perceived seriousness of the condition. Outcome expectation of medical attention includes perceived gains from what is done, perceived obstacles to doing it, and effectiveness prospects.

Self-efficacy theory

(Bandura, 1977) – Clarifies human actions by the vibrant, mutual interface with actions, personal elements, and surroundings.

Health promotion model

(Pender, 2002) – Actions that support health are motivated by a number of cognitive-perceptual elements like how important well-being is and the perceived gains, perceived control of well-being and self-effectiveness, and adapted by elements like demographics and interpersonal pressures.

Erikson's stages of psychosocial development

(Erikson, 1963):
- Trust vs. mistrust
- Autonomy vs. shame and doubt
- Initiative vs. guilt
- Industry vs. inferiority
- Identity vs. role confusion
- Intimacy vs. isolation
- Generativity vs. stagnation
- Ego identity vs. despair

Health behavior change models

PRECEDE model:
(Green & Kreuter, 1991) – Has to do with recognizing and evaluating the learner's quality of life and diagnosing health issues and danger elements. PRECEDE stands for: Predisposing, Reinforcing, and Enabling Causes in Educational Diagnosis and Evaluation. These elements are utilized for creating educational involvement to make alterations and policies to help these alterations occur.

Change theory:
(Lewin) – Advanced practice settings are vibrant. Arranged alterations meant that there must be an unfreezing of the current way of doing things, put the change into action, refreeze/create, then recognize and habitually utilize the new way.

Transtheoretical model:

(Prochaska & Velicer, 1997) – Came from a comparative study of more than 300 theories. The fundamental model is:

- Precontemplation
- Contemplation
- Preparation
- Action
- Maintenance

Stress

Stress is defined as the disparity between the burdens the patient carries from the surroundings and the patient's personal and community resources that are needed to handle the burden. Some stressors include key life happenings, every day aggravations, ongoing tension, devastating happenings, and ambient elements (ongoing from the surroundings, like noise irritations). Selye's 1974 theory of General Adaptation Syndrome is a continuum that shows that just a little bit of stress can be inspiring and give the patient a better life, but after the stress goes beyond a particular point it turns into a psychological and physical encumbrance. In the body, indications of stress include gastrointestinal signs, head pain, tight muscles, high blood pressure, agitation, and clammy hands. Emotionally, the signs include tetchiness, emotional bursts, sobbing, depression, withdrawal, aggression, a propensity to hold someone else at fault, worry, and suspiciousness. Actions that demonstrate stress include lassitude, not caring, no focus, bad memory, less efficiency, not showing up, and sleep problems.

Coping with stress:

Ways to lessen stress include organization of time, allowing certain amounts of time for certain things, staying away from change (in times of a lot of life alteration), making regular routines, changing the environment to lessen stressors, and getting into things that are of interest (lessens thinking about self). In the behavior, encourage the patient to raise the self-worth by being more aware of good points, more assertive, and practicing meditation or prayer. Counter-conditioning that lessens the stress reaction may be done. This includes autogenic training (repeating autogenic phrases), imagery, tension-relaxation drills, and biofeedback. Physical activity creates physiological alterations that counteract the way stress works on a patient. Stress management is much harder if the patient has significant depression, hallucinations, delusions, short-term hypotensive or hypoglycemic condition, or significant hurting. Bomar (2004) said there is a sturdy link for social support and well-being, including:

- Emotional support – Compassion, love, trust, concern, etc.
- Instrumental support – Costs, groups, noncircuitous help, etc.
- Educational support – Data, guidance, ideas, etc.
- Assessment support – Ways to self weigh how things are going, affirmation, etc.

Social support:

Pender (2002) said that social support is linked to getting well after being sick, moving on from crisis, doing well with losing weight, and more types of good life alterations. Support groups are able to give help for someone that does not have a sturdy and optimistic group of his or her own. Other studies propose that *good* support is more worthwhile than a *lot* of support and gives more of an indication of health. Relationships help shield patients from the bad outcomes that come from stressful circumstances.

Healthy nutrition principles

Eating a range of different kinds of foods, and eating increased amounts fruits, vegetables, whole grains, poultry and fish. Diets should consist of 55%–60% carbohydrates, less than 30% fat, and the rest should be protein (.8–1.0 g/kg). Restrict fat to < 30% of all calories. Restrict saturated fat to < 10%. Restrict cholesterol to 300 mg/day. Utilize moderate amounts of sugar, salt, and sodium. Look at the US Department of Agriculture's food guide pyramid. Take a multivitamin including folic acid if the patient is female and able to have children. Get 200–800 IU/day of vitamin D in order to absorb calcium. Calcium intake should be: 1300 mg/day for women age 13–18 or those who are pregnant/nursing; 1000 mg/day for women age 19–50 years; 1500 mg/day for age 51 years and older. Patients who are pregnant or having chemotherapy should not try to lose weight. There may be a need to lose weight with diabetes, joint pain, a lot of inflammation, cardiovascular disease, hypothyroidism, or renal disease.

Health screening

Broad screening for conditions that are very likely to occur and diseases that are likely to kill if they are not identified. The assessment should be trustworthy using proper techniques and proper follow-up. The assessment needs to be sensitive, with a true positive outcome when the outcome is positive, and it should be particular, with a true negative for someone that does not have the condition.

Check-ups

Adolescent:
(Ages 12–19 years) check-ups – According to the American Medical Association (AMA), an adolescent also needs 3 regular checks at ages 11–14, 15–17, then 18–21 years, except when more visits are needed. When there is a big chance, give advice and assess for HIV and VDRL, and check understanding of birth control and condoms. Immunizations include Tetanus-diphtheria booster and more when necessary. Be aware of indications of depression or suicide. Get a dental exam every year. For girls, instruct about self-breast exam, identify Tanner stage (regarding puberty), and do Pap smear if over the patient is having sex or is over the age of 18 years. Tanner stages include:
- Stage I – Growth spurt (average age 10).
- Stage II – Breast bud; slight pubic hair.
- Stages III–IV – Breasts grow.
- Stage V – Mature.

For boys, educate regarding self-testicular exam and find Tanner stage:

- Stage I – Growth spurt (average 12 ½).
- Stage II – Minimal pubic hair.
- Stages III–IV – Penis grows larger.
- Stage V – Mature.

Young adult:

(Ages 20–39 years) – Do a total physical at 20 (5–6-year increments). Check blood pressure (2 years apart) to look for normal systolic: 110–130 mm Hg and diastolic 60–80 mm Hg. Check total cholesterol in 5-year increments and do more when it is higher than 200 mg/dL. Do PPD when patient had contact with TB, get Td immunization in 10-year increments, teach self-skin assessment, and dental check-up should occur every year. Men need to perform self- testicular exam every month. Women need self-breast exam every month, Pap and pelvic assessments in 3-year increments, GC and Chlamydia assessments, and clinical breast exam in 3-year increments.

Adults:

Adults should have these screenings:
- Blood pressure (2 years apart).
- Cholesterol (5 years apart).
- Dental (yearly).
- ECG (over 40, yearly when there are cardiac risks).
- Pap smear (female over 18, 3 years apart following two fine outcomes and no risks).
- Self breast exam (over 20, monthly).
- Clinical breast exam (over 40, yearly; 20-39 3 years apart).
- Mammogram (over 40, yearly; some say 1-2 years apart).
- Colorectal screen (over 50, yearly).
- Prostate-specific antigen (men over 50, yearly).
- Glaucoma (over 40, yearly when there are risks).
- Hearing (if patient has a lot of contact with noise).
- Chest x-ray (not advised).

- Thyroid palpation (20-39, 3 years apart; 40 and up, yearly).
- Urinalysis (debatable).
- Hgb/Hct (debatable).
- Health education and promotion (every time patient is seen).

Middle-age check-up:

(Ages 40–59) – Get a total physical (5–6 years apart), check blood pressure (2 years apart) to see normal systolic: 110–130 mm Hg and diastolic 60–80 mm Hg. The aim is < 120/80 if the patient has diabetes or ongoing renal problem. Check cholesterol (5 years apart) and do more when it is > 200 mg/dL. Do ECG at 40 years and older when there is a chance of cardiac problems. Women need self-breast exam every month, clinical breast exam every year, ACS says mammogram every year (USPSTF says 1–2 years apart), and Pap and pelvic assessment (3 years apart when there are not any other risks). Men need STE every month. All middle-age adults need colorectal screen at age 50 (yearly), glaucoma screen (yearly), dental assessment and cleaning (6–12 months apart), cancer screen (every year) and tetanus (10 years apart).

Exams:

Evaluation of rectum and prostate: Ask the male patient to bend forward over the table so that the chest and shoulders are relaxed on it. If the man is not able to get up from lying down, use the left lateral Sims' position so that the right knee is bent and the left leg is stretched out.

Evaluation of scrotum for a fully grown Hispanic male: Hispanic male – The sac will be unbalanced so that the left side is lower than the right. The sac will be a darker shade than the rest of the patient's skin. In someone with red hair, the sac will have a reddish shade. If there is a reddish shade without red hair, there may be a problem. The sac is covered in material that can be coarse, and there can be little skin bumps that are actually sebaceous or epidermoid cysts. These cysts might give an oily emission.

Elderly check-up:

Get a total physical (2 years apart) including lab tests, check blood pressure (2 years apart) to see: normal systolic 110–120 mm Hg, diastolic 60–80mm Hg. Check total cholesterol (5 years apart) and do more when it is over 200 mg/dL. Do ECG every year when there are cardiac risks. Women need self-breast exam every month, mammogram (ACS says every year; USPSTF says 1–2 years apart), and Pap and pelvic assessment (3 years apart). Men need self-testicular exam every month. Everyone needs colorectal screen (fecal occult or sigmoidoscopy) at age 50 (yearly), glaucoma test (yearly), dental exam and cleaning (6–12 months apart), tetanus shot (10 years apart) pneumococcal vaccine (one time) and influenza vaccine (every year). Top reasons elderly die include: heart disease, cerebrovascular disease, obstructive lung disease, pneumonia and/or influenza, lung cancer, colorectal cancer.

Adolescents

Adolescents (age 12–19) – Top reasons adolescents die: car wrecks, suicide, accidents, malignancy, cardiovascular disease, congenital disease. Expect alterations in the body with puberty and a necessity for taking responsibility for well-being, diet, physical activity, getting enough sleep, and staying out of danger. Eat a range of food and eat breakfast, good snacks, and restrict sugar and fast food. Take care of the skin. Take care of the dental needs, including using fluoride and going to the dentist (6–12 months apart). Keep safe: wear protective gear when doing sports, seat belts, gun safety, defensive driving, coaching about driving, and stay away from aggressive actions or gangs. The adolescent will need habitual exercise with sports, social life, and being active in school and/or church. Do not smoke or stop smoking, and make a point about how it makes the patient become unattractive (teeth and nails, bad breath, clothes smell) and do worse in sports (cannot go as long; lose breath easily). Sexuality issues include dating, being accountable for sex life, abstinence, birth control, and chances of STDs or unplanned pregnancy.

Adolescent physical:

Utilize anthropometric chart for height and weight. Assess for an eating disorder when needed. Evaluate the patient's point of view about eating and body weight. Check the skin. Look for gingivitis, caries, and problems with alignment. Check for indications of abuse or neglect. If the patient has been near a lot of noise, check the hearing. Check sight. Check the blood pressure (2 years apart) to see normal at 120/80 mm Hg or lower. Do a TB skin assessment (2 years apart), if there has been any contact or if the patient has a chance of getting TB.

Young adults

Young adults (ages 20–39) – Top reasons for death include car wrecks, murder, suicide, harm to the body, heart disease, and AIDS. As far as eating and physical activity, the patient needs to maintain a healthy weight (even with adjustments in the basal metabolic rate) and choose a routine of physical activity. Get proper dental work. Regarding sexuality, make arrangements for planning the family or birth control and avoiding STDs. Educate regarding signs of cancer and taking care of the skin. Stop smoking as the main way to prevent problems, and educate regarding drinking alcohol or using other substances. The patient needs to keep safe by using protective gear in sports or exercise, seat belts, helmets, practicing gun safety, driving carefully, and avoiding aggressive actions. The patient will need coping mechanisms for stress and family and parenting abilities. Be aware of personal well being with regard to protection and the surroundings.

Middle-age patients

Middle-age patients (ages 40–59) – Top reasons for death include heart disease, accidents, lung cancer, cerebrovascular disease, breast cancer, colorectal cancer, and obstructive lung disease. As far as eating and physical activity, the patient needs to maintain a healthy weight (even with adjustments in the basal metabolic rate) and choose a routine of physical activity. Get proper dental work. Deal with menopause, sexual alterations that come with getting older,

STDs, indications of cancer, and taking care of the skin. Stop smoking as the main way to prevent problems, and educate regarding drinking alcohol or using other substances. The patient needs to keep safe by using protective gear in sports or exercise, seat belts, helmets, practicing gun safety, driving carefully, and avoiding aggressive actions. Deal with mid-life issues, including children leaving home, becoming grandparents, getting ready for retirement, and coping with stress. Be aware of personal well-being with regard to protection and the surroundings.

Elderly patients

Elderly (ages 60 and older) – Top reasons for death include heart disease, cerebrovascular disease, obstructive lung disease, pneumonia and/or influenza, lung cancer, and colorectal cancer. As far as eating and physical activity, the patient needs to maintain a healthy weight (even with adjustments in the basal metabolic rate) and choose a routine of physical activity. Get proper dental work. Deal with sexual differences that occur because of getting older and any STDs. Look for cancer indications and take care of the skin. Stop smoking as the main way to prevent problems, and educate regarding drinking alcohol or using other substances. The patient needs to keep safe by using protective gear in sports or exercise, seat belts, helmets, practicing gun safety, driving carefully, and avoiding aggressive actions. Deal with differences in the way life is, including retirement, losing a husband, wife, or friends, and dealing with differences in the body (sight, hearing, responses, bowel/bladder routines). Be aware of personal well-being with regard to protection and the surroundings.

Centers for Disease Control and Prevention plans

<u>Hepatitis B vaccine:</u>
3-dose routing is encouraged for everyone at newborn, 1–2 months, and 4–6 months. Fully grown patients who have a higher risk of getting it are patients in healthcare jobs, patients that have a likelihood of blood or blood product exposure, and patients increase their risk with sexual intercourse. Use serologic assessments to find out when and whether periodic

boosters are necessary. If the patient did not get the immunization as a youth, they should get this vaccine.

Tetanus-diphtheria vaccine:

Main series is advised it if was not done as a child, including 2 doses that are a minimum of 4 weeks away from each other and the third dose 6–12 months following that. The Td booster is encouraged (10 years apart). At age 14–16, a booster should be administered when it has not been done within 5 years before that.

Measles-mumps-rubella vaccine:

Encouraged for adolescents who did not get two doses when they were 12 months old or after that. The second dose should be administered routinely during the preschool immunizations or when the patient is 12–14 years old, or before postsecondary instruction or going into the military. Fully grown patients who do not have records of disease or immunization have a necessity of just one dose. Patients with a birthday before 1956 are thought to be immune.

Varicella vaccine:

Encouraged for patients who never experienced the chicken pox. Youth and fully grown patients will get 2 doses that are 4–8 weeks away from each other.

Influenza vaccine:

Encouraged as a yearly event for fully grown patients and kids who have ongoing problems with lung and cardiovascular systems (asthma, diabetes, renal problems), patients 50 years of age or older, and anyone who has an ongoing health problem. Patients who may give influenza to others that are in high-risk groups (work in health care or live in same house with high risk patient) need to get this immunization. The best time to get it is the middle of October through the middle of November. Do NOT get it with prior anaphylactic hypersensitivity to eggs or another element. See a doctor to get the right treatment and judge any allergy issues.

Hepatitis A vaccine:

Give 2 doses at newborn and 6–12 months for patients who have jobs in or are going to places that have a lot of HAV infection cases, gay men, patients who use parenteral drugs, have been in contact with non-human primates, or have ongoing liver disease.

Polio:
Inactivated poliovirus vaccine-enhanced potency (IVP-e) – Needed for any fully-grown patient who has not been immunized and is going to a country outside the United States or works in a healthcare job. Someone who has been partly immunized or has not been immunized and has exposure to kids getting OPV should get this immunization. The second dose should be administered a month after the initial one. The third is given 6 months after that.

Lyme disease:
Given to patients who are 15 years of age or older who have jobs in endemic geographic regions since they have more danger of this condition.

Unclear immunization records

Use this schedule for patients with unclear immunization records – The first time, get Td, IPV, MMR, and HBV. Elective immunizations that are chosen due to risk elements include HAV, varicella, influenza, and pneumococcal. The next time, which should occur in 4–6 weeks, get Td, IPV, and HBV. If these were done on the first visit, get the next dose of HAV and varicella. The last time happens 6 months later, and includes Td, IPV, HBV, and a third dose of HAV for children.

Clear records of childhood vaccines

Youth and fully grown patients should get hepatitis B series, Td booster (10 years apart), varicella (when necessary) given in 2 doses that are 4–8 weeks away from each other, and

MMR when the patient's date of birth is after 1956. Patients who are older than 65, have ongoing disease, or live with people with ongoing diseases (heart, lung, diabetes), should get influenza vaccines every year and pneumococcal vaccine.

Immunizations not recommended

Should not be given if there is an anaphylactic response to a recognized element with these:
- MMR and influenza – Eggs
- Hepatitis – Bakers yeast
- IPV – Streptomycin, polymyxin B, neomycin
- Varicella – Gelatin, neomycin

Do not give immunizations if the patient has a medium or significant sickness with a high body temperature that is> 100.4°. Do not give live virus to anyone that is immunocompromised. For MMR, the patient should not get pregnant for 3 months after getting it.

Walking up steps with crutches

The leg that is unharmed should step up first. Bring up the crutches and hurt leg second. That way the weight is put on the leg that is unharmed and the crutches will bear up the hurt one.

Quadriceps setting

Elevate the foot, and push the thigh down toward the floor. Stay that way for 5 seconds.

Exercises

Straight leg raise:

Raise one stretched out leg when sitting down on the floor. Sit back to lean on the elbows. The other leg should be bent (90°). This is used to strengthen the quadriceps and is good for someone with patellofemoral stress syndrome.

Terminal arc extension:

Lie down on the back, on the floor. Bend the knees slightly (20°) and put a rolled towel under the knees. Straighten a leg out and keep it straight for 5 seconds. This is used to strengthen the quadriceps and is good for someone with patellofemoral stress syndrome.

Health screenings

Child with JRA:

Habitual screening for ulcerative colitis, diabetes mellitus, and adrenal insufficiency are needed.

Someone at risk for colon cancer:

Fecal occult blood assessment, flexible sigmoidoscopy. The first indication of colon cancer is guaiac positive stool, which is found using the Hemoccult assessment. Fecal occult blood assessment is the way to get and assess six samples using 3 consecutive stools that are taken from the patient's home. Flexible sigmoidoscopy lets you have noncircuitous sight to assess the distal portions of the colon and rectum. This is done by a trained examiner by way of the flexible endoscope after cleaning the descending and sigmoid colon and rectum. It can find 80% of neoplasms found in the colorectal region. American Cancer Society (2001) advises the fecal occult blood test every year and sigmoidoscopy tests 5 years apart for anyone over 50. Any positive outcome needs to be further looked at with a colonoscopy. The colonoscopy lets you see the whole colon and rectum.

Growth and development

Long bones, myelinization, and differentiation of the central nervous system continue until a patient turns 25 years of age. After that, a patient might grow 1/8 to 1/4 of an inch taller (males more than females). Female's skulls are more likely to get bigger than males. There are some bones that keep getting longer during the lifespan. The muscles keep getting stronger and are at their strongest from age 25 to 30 years. The heart does not get bigger with aging, so if a patient has a bigger-than-normal heart, it is a cardiac problem. A dilated left ventricle happens if there is a heart attack, while different cardiac functioning happens due to cardiac disease.

Vision in middle age

In middle age, the eyes change. The pupils do not adjust as easily when moving from an area with good light to an area that is dark. This is because the pupils are smaller due to getting older. The muscles are weaker.

Tinetti Balance and Gait Evaluation

Used to assess the balance and gait issues that elderly patients have. The patient has to do certain things, such as sitting down and standing up from a chair, turning around, bending over, and other things. The entire assessment takes approximately 15– 20 minutes. The Up-and-Go assessment is another choice. A more complicated one is the Lawton and Brody: Instrumental Activities of Daily Learning, and is used to check whether the patient can do more complicated things like go shopping, wash clothes, cook, and more. The Index of Independence of Activities of Daily Living is utilized to find what the patient can do for themselves on a regular basis.

Adjustments with aging

<u>Life events:</u>
Holmes and Rahe Social Readjustment Rating Scale says that the most adjustment happens after a husband or wife dies. Other major life events also require adjustment, including ending a marriage, getting separated from a spouse, or losing a job.

<u>Iron absorption:</u>
As one ages, it is common for there to be less iron absorption. The thyroid gland generally stays the same, but getting older could cause there to be fibrosis and more nodularity. Other differences with aging in the GI system include an increase in adipose tissue, smaller liver, less motility and peristalsis, less acid secretions, and motor work in the stomach, and less glomerular filtration.

<u>Senile lentigines:</u>
A shade of gray/brown, these are asymmetrical, macular lesions that show up on areas that have been in the sun. It is common to see them on the face, arms, and hands. It occurs with aging.

<u>Romberg's sign:</u>
Shows that a patient cannot keep their balance. When someone has this, they require more assessments.

Issues with the elderly

<u>Driving:</u>
An elderly patient has differences in the senses. Lessened ability to hear does not mean a patient cannot drive, but sight is very important, including binocular sight, ability to see color, and ability to see in the dark.

REM:
Rapid eye movement starts approximately 120 minutes after going to sleep, and happens again in 3–4 evenly spread out increments that last 10–15 minutes. It is linked to skeletal muscle atonia, rapid eye movements, and dreaming. It happens less as one gets older. With aging, the patient is more likely to wake up, and there is more sleep latency. Sleep is not as good in an older patient. Even though more time is given to lying in bed, the actual time asleep is not as much.

Immunity:
Not as strong as aging occurs, therefore an older patient is more likely to get an infection. There is not as much thymus-gained immunity because the thymus gland is smaller. This also means it is harder for an older patient to make antibodies.

Incontinence:
There is not as strong of a bladder, less ability to concentrate urine, and less urethral closing pressure following menopause. These factors cause incontinence. Incontinence is also influenced by depression, less ability to move, less ability to see, and not as much focus on feeling a full bladder.

Antibodies:
An elderly patient can react to an infection with antibodies that have been created by the body before, but if the problem is new, it is more difficult. Cells in the immune system cannot proliferate as easily in an older patient as in a younger one. The amount of T-cells is stable, but they do not work as well and can have less cytotoxicity.

Allergies:
Find out what kind of response the patient has with an allergy, especially when getting the patient history. Determine if the response is actually an allergy to a medication or actually an adverse effect of it.

Screening for prostate cancer

The advised schedule starts when the man turns 40 and includes digital-rectal exam (DRE). Start PSA assessments when the patient is 50 unless there are reasons to initiate sooner. Although the urinalysis and complete blood count (CBC) will be done in a regular yearly evaluation, they are not used to screen for this condition. Do PSA and DRA for a male that is older than 50.

Alendronate

Patient education:
Alendronate (Fosamax) – Take it with a whole glass of water when you first wake up, half-an-hour prior to breakfast. Stay upright after taking it so that the esophagus will not be influenced. If you take it with food, the bioavailability goes down 40%. If you take it with coffee or orange juice, bioavailability goes down 60%. If you take it after breakfast, the amount absorbed decreases considerably.

Skipped oral contraceptives

If an oral contraceptive has been missed for several days, encourage the patient to keep up with taking the pills, and tell her that she should use an additional, alternate type of birth control for the remainder of the cycle.

Diaphragm

It can be inserted a maximum of 2 hours before having sex. It must not be removed before 6 hours have gone by after finishing having sex. It should not be worn for more than 24 hours.

Breast self-exam

<u>Implants:</u>

Educate the patient on the fact that she still needs to do the BSE every month. Mammography is not sufficient by itself. Review how to do it with the patient until she can do it easily, including what to feel for with the new implants.

Nurse Practitioner and Patient Relationship

Health assessment

Get an account of prior health issues so that you will know what activities give the patient more of a chance of problems and you will be able to give the proper instruction for that patient. The health history should include demographics and biographical information. It should include an account of current health problems, including the OPQRST assessment:

- Onset
- Provocative/palliative (getting well or problem going downhill)
- Quality/quantity
- Region/radiation
- Setting
- Timing

Find out about prior health issues, including how the patient feels he is generally doing, prior conditions or times in the hospital, harm or operations (including when, what the medical attention was, and what check-ups were done afterwards), emotional well-being, sexual well-being, allergies to food or drugs (and the particular problem that happens including needed medical attention for it if there is any), drugs (prescribed and over-the-counter), immunizations (when and what), sleep routines, and prior assessments for any part of the body. Discuss individual routines, including the utilization of tobacco, alcohol, drugs, caffeine, nutrition, physical activity, hobbies, athletics, and contact sports.

Relative's health issues:

Talk about relatives, including how old they are, how mom and dad's health is or why they died, well-being of sisters and brothers, health of children, and any conditions that are hereditary.

Athletics:

Discuss any restrictions from athletics, rapid heart rate or chest hurting upon physical activity, seizure, concussion, prior loss of consciousness, whether the patient can run for a half- mile (or higher), and whether the patient has both kidneys.

Psychosocial factors:

Find out about the patient's psychosocial factors, including where he currently lives, what level of schooling he has finished (or what grade he is currently in if it is an adolescent, including how his grades are and how the school experience is going), faith (as it relates to well-being and medical attention), his point of view of a normal day, optimistic or pessimistic prospects for what is to come, stress and coping mechanisms, depression, anxiety, or thoughts of suicide. Teens and young adults should be asked straight out, as in, "Have you ever thought about ending your own life?" Ask about the social network.

Work and surroundings:

Get an account of the patient's work and the atmosphere where they spend time. Find out what kind of job they have, prior jobs, any dangerous contact with anything at home or on the job, time in the military or in a war (when applicable), where the patient lives and how long they have lived there, whether the home is anywhere near a factory, shipyard, or another thing that could have harmful elements, and find out about leisure pursuits and any other possible contact with unsafe elements.

Adolescents:

If the patient is an adolescent, let them be the one to give the account, and let them know that except when the issue becomes significant or puts their life in danger, the account is private. A broadly used system for getting a medical history from an adolescent is HEADSS: Home, Education, Activities, Drugs, Sex, and Suicide. This model includes age-appropriate direction.

Finding risk factors

Find out risk factors, as almost every health problem comes with risk elements.

Research:

Research from the last 20 years demonstrates that there are certain elements that are linked to well-being and having a longer, quality lifespan. These include physical activity, not smoking (current research also expands this to staying in smoke-free surroundings), sleeping for 7–8 hours a night, sensible or no consumption of alcohol, eating regularly in sensible amounts with breakfast as one of the meals, and maintaining a healthy weight. Plenty of physical activity, eating well, and healthy living will slow the aging progression.

Cardiac:

Cardiac risk elements include: man that is 45 years of age or older; woman who is 55 years of age or older or in early menopause, relatives who have had early heart disease or heart attack, father who died younger than 55 or mom who died younger than 65 years of age. More cardiac elements include: smoking, hypertension, or taking antihypertensive drugs, diabetes mellitus, low HDL cholesterol < 35 mg/dL (but > 60 mg/dL gives a negative risk), and LDL > 160 mg/dL (but < 130 mL gives a negative risk).

Obesity:

Obesity is when a patient is at least 20% over the desired weight. The chance of death increases when the patient weights 10% more than desired weight, and obesity is linked to many other health risks. Someone with hypertension or type 2 diabetes is 3 times more likely to be obese. There is more of a chance of high cholesterol, coronary artery disease, and these types of cancer: colon, rectal, prostate, gallbladder, biliary tract, breast, cervical, endometrial, and ovarian. Abdominal adiposity is linked to more chance of stroke and dying for any reason.

Suicide:

Suicide risks include relatives who have had psychiatric problems (particularly depression or suicide), prior times of trying to kill oneself, aggression in the family (verbal, bodily, or sexual abuse), unbalanced home life (ongoing separation or losing someone that is loved), misuse of alcohol or another substance, and being able to get to a firearm inside the residence.

Interviewing an elderly patient

Care vs. cure: get better or preserve the patient's quality of life. Get a total and truthful account of the patient's medical history in the form of a personal account. A lot of the data gathered can be used to identify what the problem is and what the medical treatment will be. Build up the relationship with the patient by creating an atmosphere of trust and compassion. Find out what the main grievance is. Keep the interview focused on the aim because the patient might come in with a lengthy, complicated medical past. Control the dialogue, but stay away from a positive review (where the patient merely has to say yes to each query). Go over each matter separately. The patient's gender and how old he/she is can be a factor in the relationship. Other family members can help, and the patient might depend on them to help answer queries. Delicate matters like incontinence, abuse, failing mental ability, or sexual difficulties should be discussed. It is important to make the patient know that the discussion is confidential.

Communication and environment:

Do not talk fast. Use a low tone in your voice so that the patient can hear you better. Aid the patient in illuminating what he or she might be feeling, and get them to verify this. Express kindness and connection by paying attention and the use of suitable physical contact. Watch for indications of stress, tiredness, or uneasiness. Try to comprehend social backgrounds, ethnic differences, language issues, or individual partialities. Make sure the conversation is in a soothing environment, where no one can overhear. Put a restriction on how long the interview goes because an aged patient gets tired faster. Talk facing each other so that you can meet the patient's eyes. Be calm but concerned. Make sure there is good lighting and air, and make sure the light does not come from in back of you (to avoid shadowing or shining in the eyes).

Health history:

Biographical information, family background regarding medical histories, job, drugs being used, use of cigarettes, use of drugs that are against the law, allergies, problems with drugs or foods, mental problems, diet, sleep, physical activity, leisure activities, overview of systems, and prevention being done (such as screenings). Get an account of the prior medical treatment, including any time the patient had to go to the hospital, surgeries, vaccinations, accidents, harm done, falling down, medical conditions from the past (including as a kid), communicable diseases from the past, health practices, and religious elements that influence the body (such as fasting). Check into safety concerns including work, home, and other places, the ability to drive, or any abuse. Discuss the Patient Self-Determination Act from 1990, including any advance directives, a living will, power of attorney, and doctor-assisted suicide. Find out where and with whom the patient lives, including who the main caregiver is. Talk about how a disability will affect income, and discuss help that can be found in the area.

Professional Role and Policy

National Council of State Boards of Nursing

Advanced practice registered nursing:

According to the NCSBN, an advanced practice registered nurse is acting as a nurse with a foundation on information and proficiency that was obtained in basic nursing school; has a license to be an RN and has completed and received a diploma from graduate school in an APRN program that has been accredited from a nationwide accrediting body; has up-to-date certification from a nationwide certification board to work in the proper APRN area. Being an APRN defines the nurse as someone that has more responsibility, which may or may not come with more pay or gain for the nurse.

Some responsibilities include:
- Give professional education and leadership.
- Handle patient and medical center leadership.
- Support the patient and local area by keeping the ideal concerns for the patient or community.
- Assess reactions of involvement and how well medical routines are working.
- Be in touch with and act together with patients, patient relatives, and colleagues.
- Employ research; get and use new information and equipment.
- Educate others regarding APRN.
- Evaluate the patient, produce and assess information; comprehend higher nursing practice in action at this rank.
- Assess many kinds of information; find differential diagnosis; determine proper medical care.
- Without supervision, determine how to handle difficult patient issues.
- Create a way to identify the condition, create objectives for the patient's medical management, and stipulate the medical routine or plan.

- Identify, set the routine for medical management, oversee, and give out the medical plan. This includes medicine and drugs as appropriate that fall inside of the APRN's area.
- Handle the patient's bodily and mental condition.
- Make sure there is protected and pertinent nursing being done, whether direct or indirect with regard to the patient.
- Keep protected and beneficial surroundings.

APRN positions:

Advanced practice registered nurse (APRN) – Includes nurse anesthetists, nurse midwives, nurse practitioners, and clinical nurse specialists. These must have proper credentials and take the role of the main leadership in taking responsibility for the patient's care. Some other patients who hold leadership responsibilities are not included under the term APRN. These patients who are not included may have professional responsibilities but not in a clinical setting, such as teachers, administrators, or researchers, even though these patients may have the same knowledge as an APRN. Someone that is not working in a client or family medical clinic cannot be an APRN. More than the 2–4 years of study that is needed to become a basic nurse is required to be an APRN. The APRN will have further study to meet the extra standards.

Practice:

Leads the medical management of patients, supports the patient, is responsible for the patient goals and expense of care, medically handles patient conditions, dispenses information, leads, studies, gives advice, handles cases, and is a facilitator of modification.

Standards of practice: These are defined by the ANA (from 1998) and meant to be professional guidelines regarding the excellence of performance, service, and learning. They give the least amount of satisfactory work. It gives clients a way to determine the quality of the treatment that was given to them. There are broad and particular standards to the area of expertise. Some particular areas of expertise have their own standards as well, such as National

Association of Pediatric Nursing Practitioners (NAPNP) and Association for Women's Health, Obstetric, and Neonatal Nurses (AWHONN). PNP has separate standards. All standards may be used in legal proceedings, but they are not originally meant for this purpose.

Scope of practice: It is dependent on each state and what the patient in this position can do beneath the Nurse Practice Act for that state. The scope gives guidelines instead of particular directives. There is a big range, depending on the state. Many times the scope is founded on what is allowed legally both in the state and in the nation. The initial Scope of Practice for PNPs occurred in 1983 by the National Association of Pediatric Nurse Practitioners. This has been updated in 1990 and in 2000. Scope is always changing and improving.

Multistate licensure compact: From 1998, 17 states have decided to pass legislation so that RN licenses are acknowledged in the states that choose to take part. Wisconsin was the initial state (in 2000) to allow APRNs to take part as well inside of the legislation dealing with this issue. In 2000, a position paper was written by NCSBN and NP stakeholders to deal with how to handle multistate acknowledgement of ARPN licenses and ability to do work.

Clinical privileges: 1983: The chance of hospital staff membership became an opportunity for people who were not doctors by the joint Commission on Accreditation of Health Care Organizations (JCAHO). This subject matter is still in progress.

Nursing practice acts

See the NCSBN Web site to find the complete list of state practice acts (not for every state, but 31 states are included): http://www.nesbn.org. An authorizing board of nursing is available in every state to lead statutes with regard to licenses for an RN. They have responsibility for how titles are used, scope of work, and how to handle discipline cases. Nurse practice acts come out of statutory law.

Pediatric nurse practitioner

(PNP) – According to the National Association of Pediatric Nurse Practitioners, the PNP has the education to be an APRN and uses the knowledge and expertise to medically treat children and young adults. To have the right credentials, the PNP has to finish a degreed program with an expertise in pediatric health care. The criteria for the State Board of Registered Nurses must be met. Some of the class subjects that are required are:
- Growth and development.
- Pathophysiology.
- Physical, developmental, family and cultural assessment.
- Lab work.
- Identification and medical handling of frequently seen sicknesses from childhood, including behavioral issues.

Nurse practitioner education

Most require a master's level education. The difference from NP to CNS is not very clear. Some master's programs now have a blended NP/CNS programs. The pros and cons of such a blended program are still being debated. The majority of NP education programs stipulate that the student complete 2 years of full-time or 3–4 years of part-time schooling.

Curriculum guidelines:

These guidelines are updated from time to time. The Association of Faculties of Pediatric Nurse Practitioner and Associate Programs (AFPNP/AP) began with the initial printed guidelines in 1981 and came out with a new edition in 1996. The National Association of Nurse Practitioner Faculties (NONPF) put out a written curriculum plan for nurse practitioners in 1990 and came out with a new edition in 1995. The basic graduate nurse has to complete the basic courses. An advanced practice RN has to complete the basic advanced courses. Each APRN will take classes that are distinctive to the kind of APRN that will be his/her specialty in order to better serve the patients. Theoretical study for the APRN includes Benner's model of expert practice from 1985, Calkin's model of advanced nursing practice from 1984, and Shuler's model of NP practice from 1993 and again updated in 1998.

Clinical practice guiding principles and practice:

These are needed so that the NP and the patient will know what is suitable with regard to medical treatment. It is different from state to state because of the different nurse practice acts for the states. Publications and notable references may be used to determine protocol needs. For instance, in pediatric care, with regard to guidelines for prevention of medical conditions, guidelines include Bright Futures (MCHB), Guidelines for Adolescent Preventative Services (AMA) and Guide to Preventative Services. As examples for pediatric care guidelines for sicknesses, there are Asthma (NIH, AAP), Hearing Screening (NIH, AAP), HIV (AHRQ), Otitis media including effusion (AHRQ), Pain (AHRQ), and Sickle Cell disease (AHRQ).

APRN credentials

- Make sure there is answerability and conscientiousness for proficient work.
- Authenticates that the patient has received the correct instruction, has a license, and is certified.
- Compulsory to make sure that the local and national laws are followed.
- Recognizes the furthered scope for the APRN.
- Allows for needed ways for patients to make a grievance.

- Allows for responsibility for the community by making sure standards of practice are met.
- Debates between the State boards of Nursing and different education accrediting organizations were more heated in the 1990s due to more NP programs coming available.
- National task force with regard to the excellence of NP schools met in 1995. Many organizations were present.
- The government does not have a hand in credentialing.
- Credentials may be obtained through an NCAA-acknowledged certifying body.

Certification for APRN

The government has no responsibility for certification. An agency or group verifies that the patient has a license and has finished specific, set-forth standards as must be met in the particular area of expertise. It might be necessary to receive a state license or reimbursement. It is necessary to become an APRN in certain states.

Writing prescriptions

NPs and Certified Nurse-Midwives (CNM) have had the ability to write certain prescriptions since the mid-1970s. Since 1998, every state allows a degree of ability to write prescriptions, although Illinois is still waiting for statutory authority. It is necessary pharmacology instruction must be included in the master's degree; the APRN has to get continued instruction to keep the authority to write prescriptions. Certain guidelines differ between the states. The range of what prescriptions are allowed is different between the states. Total ability for prescriptions includes the capability to get a federal DEA registration number.

Practice issues

Practice issues include collaboration, which is working together in such a way that everyone has a role and an importance in the practice. Acknowledge and know that the people sometimes work independently and sometimes together in order to fulfill the responsibility and action. People working in collaboration have shared objectives. The reason that collaboration is important is to give a better quality of medical attention to the patient and to give the patient a better result due to continuing stability and harmonization of medical attention. As an example, an interdisciplinary team works together in collaboration.

Case management

Working in collaboration to assess, make a plan, carry out the plan, synchronize, observe, and appraise medical choices and treatment plans so that the patient's requirements are met. Use communication and accessible wherewithal to get better, more economically sound results. The goal of case management is to activate, keep a check on, and manage the resources that a patient receiving care will need while handling the condition, as well as keeping the balance of good medical attention and economic sense.

Tasks involved:
Case management involves arranging good medical attention that also makes economic sense to get the best result, getting and managing the treatment, checking and assessing results, doing evaluations on the patient, choosing diagnostic assessments (lab or otherwise), prescribing proper drugs, competent communication and clinical proficiency, and giving a variety of medical care, lessening the fragmentation in treatment, improving life for both the patient receiving care and his or her family, and keeping money under control.

Some important factors linked to case management examples include customary proper utilization of tools with the goal of getting to recognized results inside a proper time table, endorsing collaboration, endorsing coordination of a variety of medical attention during the entire time the patient needs care, endorsing job contentment among workers, endorsing patient and worker contentment regarding medical attention and spending the least amount of money that is necessary to give good care.

<u>Patients needing case management:</u>

Needed for someone that requires medical attention that will be expensive and changeable, someone that has to come back to the hospital often or on an ongoing basis, or someone that has more than one provider or needs more than one type of care.

Quality improvement

Also called total quality management (TQM), and continuous quality improvement (CQI). It is not the same thing as quality assurance (QA) because it goes on all the time instead of from time to time. It is planned formation of change for the good or realization of unmatched quality of work for the first time. It is methodical and planned and involves structures, ways of doing things, and what results may be projected with regard to excellence and in order to make sure there is responsibility for how good the medical attention is. QI gives guidelines for continuing assessment of practice. This is done by knowing the norms, measure, and standards with which effectiveness is determined and by having minimizing liabilities.

<u>Accomplishing quality improvement:</u>

Accomplished through peer review or another form of assessment. In peer review, the approach is to acknowledge and prize the work nurses do. This shows the way toward better standards of work and puts off work that is not within what the practitioner can legally do. It heightens the quality of medical attention and gives a means for attaining answerability and conscientiousness. Another form of assessment may include an audit, question/answer or appraisal, or patient contentment question/answer or appraisal.

Risk management

Organizations and actions meant to acknowledge and intercede resulting in less chance of harm to a patient and ensuing claims in opposition to the medical attention workers. This is founded on the supposition that a lot of harm done to patients could be stopped from happening in the first place. Risk management is an assessment of places when legal responsibility is an issue, like patients, methods, or how accounts are maintained. Risk management also involves instruction used to lessen the chance of a problem in a recognized part.

Liability risks:

Liability risks include the medical attention giver/patient association, communication, and educated approval or permission, clinical proficiency, self-assessment for experts regarding the necessity of keeping up-to-date records, consultation and medical appointment recommendations, guidelines, standard actions, modus operandi, and management of other people.

Malpractice

Includes an expert acting wrongly, inability to do a skill (that should reasonably be expected), disloyalty during work or in a position of trust, acting against the law to the detriment of the patient, or acting in an immoral way to the detriment of the patient. Malpractice also includes alleged professional not giving medical attention and not acting with conscientiousness or taking preventative measures that someone else in the identical industry would give to the patient to stop someone from becoming harmed. Negligence is not doing what a sensible patient would do so in a case where a patient is harmed due to this inaction.

Malpractice insurance:

This will not shield an APRN from being liable for giving medical attention with no license to do so in a case where the APRN is acting beyond what he or she is legally allowed to do in the particular state. The National Practitioner Data Bank gathers data regarding actions in opposition to medical professionals. Nurses are included in the data bank. Malpractice insurance may be occurrence coverage or claims-made coverage. Occurrence coverage is for an instance that happened when the policy was in effect, even if the date of discovery or the claim was filed after a point when the coverage ended. Claims-made coverage is for claims made inside the time that the policy was in effect, even if the instance happened at another time. Optional tail coverage contract makes the coverage go even further on a claims-made policy so that any subsequent claims that may come up as time goes by are covered even if the basic claims-made coverage time is over.

Malpractice reimbursement:

An APRN has to be reimbursed. It does not make a difference if the APRN works alone, has a joint practice together, works in a hospital, or works in managed care. Many times federal policies for Medicaid or Medicare are used to find out what the pay will be for private-pay insurance. Although the federal government includes directives that promote paying the medical worker (who is not a doctor) in a noncircuitous manner, it is common to find that there are obstacles due to state rules and regulations.

Medicaid

1965 Title XIX Social Security Act allowed for Medicaid. It is a federal/state matching plan, and federal is in charge of supervision. The money for it comes from federal and state taxes, and 50%–83% is funded by federal. Each state is able to put more services on the list and they may put restrictions (to a point) on federally directed aid. Patients who get Medicaid cannot get a bill for the aid, but states are able to give them small co-payments or deductibles for particular types of help.

Patients covered:

Although Medicaid does not provide for everyone that lives under the federal poverty rate, some patients have to be covered under the federal government rules. These patients include:
- Patients who have gotten Aid to Families with Dependent Children (AFDC) (each state makes its own criterion for this).

- Patients that are older than 65, sightless, or have complete disability can get monetary help because of the Federal Supplemental Security income (SSI).
- Pregnant women are covered for pregnancy –associated help; children younger than 6 years of age who live in families that are up to 133% of the federal poverty level.
- Kids born following September of 1983 that live in families at or under the federal poverty level.

Medicare

Federally directed; begun in 1965; gives health insurance to elderly patients and to patients with disabilities. The patient who is covered will get hospital, doctor, and further medical attention as needed. The amount that a patient makes is not a factor for eligibility. The two types are Medicare Part A and Medicare Part B – Supplementary Medical Insurance (SMI).

Medicare Part A:
Anyone 65 years of age or older that is eligible to get Social Security is automatically enrolled even if still working. Patients are able to get Social Security if they or their spouse put money into the system by way of working for at least 40 quarters. If the patient has less than 40 quarters of work, Medicare Part A requires a payment each month. If the patient is not yet 65 but has a complete disability which will be there for the rest of their life, Medicare Part A can be used after receiving Social Security benefits for 2 years. A patient with ongoing renal disease who needs either dialysis or transplant can become eligible for Part A without waiting for 2 years.

Coverages: Includes partial expenses for hospitalization, partial skilled nursing home expenses, and does not include custodial care. For home health, all of skilled care is covered, 80% of approved expenses for medical paraphernalia are covered, and hospice is generally totally covered. Hospitalization costs are determined by the anticipated expense of treatment for someone who has that particular issue. Every Medicare-covered patient who goes into the hospital becomes categorized by the diagnosis-related group (DRG). After that, the hospital gets payment for a preset sum for everyone who comes in with that particular DRG. When the expenses go beyond that, the hospital has to cover the extra expense. If the expenses are below that, the hospital gets to retain a certain percent of the extra money. An APRN will not be given money directly for working inside of a hospital.

Medicare Part B:
The patient has to pay by the month. There are some who have a low enough salary that are entitled to have this month-to-month payment be paid by Medicaid. This program is paid for by general federal revenue and by these month-to-month payments. The program covers 80% of the authorized expense for any medical attention that is required (following a yearly deductible). This includes doctor visits, physical therapy, occupational therapy, speech therapy, medical paraphernalia, assessments, and certain types of prevention treatments like Pap smears, mammograms, and hepatitis B, pneumococcal, and influenza vaccinations.

"Incident to" bills:
"Incident to" – If the APRN does "incident to" work, the invoice is given to Medicare by the doctor that has hired the APRN, and it has to be in the doctor's name with that provider number and CPT code. This will be paid with a total doctor amount and the money comes to the doctor or to the doctor's practice.

"Incident to": With regard to the work done which is essential but incidental as a portion of a doctor's personal and expert work during identification of a condition or while giving medical attention for harm or a condition. The work has to happen when the patient is in the managed care of a doctor. The APRN has to be working for that doctor's group. The work has to happen while the patient is receiving medical attention from a doctor and follow-up work has to be in such a way that the doctor is a current contributor and is supervising the medical attention. Active personal management does not indicate that this doctor has to stay in the identical room with the APRN, but the doctor does have to be somewhere in that office area and accessible to help and manage during the APRN's medical attention.

APRN Medicare reimbursement:

Legislation is from 1997; APRNs get 85% of doctor fee schedules if they are sending invoices by themselves with an APRN billing number. A doctor's management is not needed. If the APRN is under a doctor's management, the doctor's practice can get the total amount of the regular doctor's invoice. This is under the "Incident to" rules. And APRN has to have a current RN license for the state in which he/she practices, and the APRN has to meet the criteria to do NP work for primary medical attention NP. There has to be a degree from a official educational facility in the proper area, and there has to include a minimum of one academic year which involves a minimum of 4 months of education in classes and a final outcome of a degree, diploma or certificate OR the person has to have productively finished an official advanced practice instructional curriculum and have worked doing this extended position for a minimum of a year inside the year and a half prior to February 8, 1978.

Skilled nursing facilities: If the APRN does work in a skilled nursing facility (SNF) or a nursing home that is in an urban region (urban regions are legally distinct), then Medicare money may be acquired. Medicare will pay reimbursements for an APRN's work done in SNF if it is not a defined rural region with a justifiable amount of payment. That expanse cannot be more than what a doctor's fee would be for work. The money is paid to the APRN's manager.

Methods of payment for APRNs

Advanced practice nurses may be paid in one of these ways:
- Fee-for-service
- Episodic
- Capitation, PPO, HMO

Medicaid and Medicare Omnibus Budget Reconciliation Act

In 1989, the Omnibus Budget Reconciliation Act (OBRA) made it obligatory for there to be Medicaid reimbursement payment to certified children and family nurse practitioners. This started on the first day of July 1990. The practitioner has to only do what is inside of the range of what is allowed in that state. The practitioner does not have to be responsible for the management of or be linked to a doctor or another medical professional. The amount to be paid is contingent upon the state, but is in the scope of 70%– 100% of the fee-for-service doctor Medicaid amount. Children and family nurse practitioners are allowed to send an invoice to Medicaid in a noncircuitous manner following getting a provider number from the Medicaid agency for the particular state. Each state can choose to make laws letting them make Medicaid reimbursements go to more categories of NP that are not found in the federal mandates.

Covered for NP services

Restricted to work that an NP is allowed to do in that state, work that the NP normally does, and work that the NP has been trained, given instruction on, and fulfilled any conditions for as determined by the Secretary of Health and Human Services. This work is covered with Part B if/when an MD or Doctor of Osteopathy did the same work it would have been under a doctor's services, when the NP is allowed under the law to do the work in that state, if the work is done in collaboration with an MD or DO, and the work would otherwise be disqualified for coverage due to a legal exclusion.

Other third parties that give compensation

- Private insurance – Will reimburse according to contract. This is particular for each state insurance commission.
- Civilian Health and Medical Program of the United States (CHAMPUS).
- Federal medical plan – Used by patients in the armed forces, their dependents that may be living beyond a time when they have died, their families, or retirees.
- Federal Employees Health Benefit Program (FEHBP).

Centers for Medicare and Medicaid Services
- Used to be called Health Care Financing and Administration (HCFA).
- Administration for many federal plans such as Medicare, Medicaid, HIPPA, CLIA, and State children's health insurance program (SCHIP).
- See http://cms.hhs.gov for more information.

Nursing's Agenda for Health Care Reform

Encourages development of health care which gives patients the ability to get to good medical attention and help without it costing too much, and it encourages continual primary care. It fundamentally asks for vital medical attention to be found for everyone and for there to be a reorganized health care system that centers on patients, well-being and conditions so that they may get medical help in familiar, easy to get to places. It advocates providing for ongoing medical needs and insurance changes so that patients can use their coverage more easily. It asks for organizational assessment on public and private sectors regarding the use of resources, lowering expenses, and getting balanced and even reimbursement for each provider.

Health policy

Movement in the direction of primary medical attention and getting prevention earlier; encourages utilization of APRNs. The main elements that control healthcare delivery are payors, insurance companies, providers, and suppliers. Legislation regarding ways to do things and politics is included in this topic.

Medical attention

May be primary health care or managed care. Managed care includes Health Maintenance Organizations (HMO), Preferred Provider Organizations (PPO) and Point of Service (POS) plans.

HIPAA

Health Insurance Portability and Accountability Act of 1996, under Public Law 104-191. This has a goal of better organization and helpfulness in the medical system, which is to be done by regulating the way that electronic communications for administrative and economic information is done. The requirements include particular transaction regulations (including code sets), security and electronic signatures, privacy and particular identifiers that also have utilization permissions for bosses, health plans and people who give medical attention.

<u>Privacy directive:</u>

Privacy directives manage how patient's Protected Health Information (PHI) is utilized and given out for times when the data might reveal who the patient is. HIPAA controlled PHI for people who work in the health profession, health plans and health care clearinghouses. The aim is to give tough Federal shields for the right to privacy and keep the best medical attention possible. All data is protected. Under this rule, there is a covered entity including the people who do the medical attention that communicate data electronically (as in billing, claims, or paying issues), health plans, and health care clearinghouses. Utilization and giving out of the protected information has to be done to the patient when he asks for it, to HHS, or to check up on or find out if the rule is being complied to. It is allowed for the patient, treatment, payment and healthcare operations (TPO), with the chance to concur or not, public policy, "incident to", restricted information set, and with permission.

<u>Individual rights:</u>
- Covered entity duties and contact name, title, or telephone to take delivery of grievances with effectual month, day, and year.
- Access, with the right to look at and get a copy of PHI in a designated record set (DRS) in an appropriate timeframe.
- Amendment, so that each patient has the right for Covered Entity amend PHI, but this can be not approved by Covered Entity even when the account is correct and finished.

- Accounting, so that the patient has the right to get a record of what information was given out from PHI for 6 years (or less) before the month, day and year that it was asked for.
- Asked for restrictions, so that the patient can ask for limitations of utilization and giving out PHI (although Covered Entity may not allow).
- Confidential communication, so that the provider has to allow and accommodate justifiable desires for PHI information that was exchanged by alternative methods and to alternative places.
- Grievances to covered Entity.
- Grievances to Secretary (HHS/OCR).

De-identification of PHI:

Taking out particular identifiers makes it so the patient cannot be known; use of statistical technique or taking out listed identifiers (like name, geography, dates, or SSN).

Administrative necessities:

Put into practice standard ways of doing things with regard to PHI that will go along with the Privacy Rule, put into practice suitable ways to maintain privacy of PHI for administrative, technical, and physical matters, make sure there is privacy education for anyone that is employed there and make and use a way to penalize anyone that does not go along with the Privacy Rule, and select someone to be formally responsible for the standards and ways of doing things and for taking any grievances. The Privacy Rule was obligatory from April 14, 2003. The Office for Civil Rights (OCR) implements it.

Grievances:

An unceremonious assessment might give resolution to the problem in total with no official assessment becoming necessary. When it does not, start the official queries. Technical help is available.

<u>Civil Monetary Penalties:</u>

It is $100 for each infringement. The most one would have to pay is $25,000 for one calendar year for every like condition or prohibition that is infringed upon. It is a criminal penalty for unlawfully giving out information, with these consequences:

- Up to $50,000 plus a year of jail time.
- Up to $100,000 plus 5 years of jail time for information given out with false pretenses.
- Up to $250,000 plus 10 years of jail time for plan to sell, transfer, or utilize the data for commercial reasons, own gain, or malevolent reasons.
- These consequences are maintained by the Department of Justice (DOJ).

ERISA

Federal law that excuses self-funded medical and additional benefit packages (employer and union) from State authority. Seven of every 10 workers in the United States are in self-insured packages. Official disputes are being done in opposition to the extent of these ERISA exceptions.

Research Utilization

Evidence-based practice

Meticulous, well-judged, and precise utilization of recent most excellent proof regarding medical attention for each patient that uses both medical know-how and patient ideals. The main types of primary research include:
- Therapy – To assess how well the medical attention is going. Random, double-blind, placebo-managed.
- Identification of conditions and screening – Takes accounts of legitimacy and dependability for assessments or assesses how well the assessment works to identify a condition before patient indications occur. Cross-sectional survey.
- Causation or harm – Checks if a substance is linked to an arising health problem. Cohort or case-managed.
- Prognosis – Predicts how the condition will turn out. Longitudinal cohort study.
- Systemic review – Synopsis of published works which utilizes particular ways to work to do a complete published works investigation and critical evaluation of particular studies; utilizes proper statistics to put the legitimate studies together.
- Meta-analysis – Methodical review; quantitative. Makes a synopsis of outcome.

Levels of strength of evidence-based practice:
- Level I (A–D) – Meta-analysis or a number of controlled studies together.
- Level II (A–D) – Individual experimental study.
- Level III (A–D) – Quasi-experimental study.
- Level IV (A–D) – Nonexperimental study.
- Level V (A–D) – Case report or methodically acquired; confirmable quality or program assessment information.
- Level VI – Judgment of esteemed authorities; also regulatory or legal opinions.

Published prevention courses of action

Courses of action are published in:
- *Put Prevention into Practice* – U.S. Public Health Service; regarding prevention for primary medical attention.
- *Clinicians Handbook of Preventive Service: Put Prevention Into Practice*, 1998 – for primary medical attention. http://www.ahcpr.gov/clinic/ppiphand.htm.
- *Guide to Clinical Preventive Services*, U.S. Preventive Services Task Force, 1996 – for both practice and instructional atmospheres.

Research for advanced practice

Research founded on practice is vital for getting better advanced practice nursing for years to come. The most important drift these days is toward outcome studies. You may find outcomes of studies at conferences, in publications, or through summaries of the studies themselves. Research may be paid for by the federal government, including:
- Agency for Healthcare Research and Quality (AHRQ) – http://www.ahcpr.gov.
- National Institutes of Health (NIH) – http://www.nih.gov.
- Maternal and Child Health Bureau (MCHB) – http://www.mchb.hrsa.gov.

<u>Utilization:</u>

Utilized for creating new research; founded clinical ways of working, to keep a record of clinical results and differences, to show excellence and ways to keep expenses down for medical attention, to create organization for demonstration tasks, and to get more excellent care and better results for the patient. For the patient, research is a good thing because it gives a better comprehension of the patient's circumstances, gives a better evaluation of the circumstances, results in more value in the medical treatment, creates a situation of more understanding for the patient's circumstance, and helps providers better identify the requirement for and success of treatment plans. The problems include time and expense, workers that do not want to make alterations, no rewards for utilizing the results of the study, and incomprehension or doubt about the research results. To deal with these problems, make an atmosphere that sees the use of and will utilize the study, make an atmosphere that encourages inquiry, rational thought and assesses nursing care, and promote research by giving enough time and money for it.

Professional organizations

They are used to set up standards of work, as a cooperative way to endorse the practice of nursing and the best medical treatment possible, to check on and give weight to policy and law issues, to put out position papers, and to educate. Some examples:
- American Nurse Association (ANA)
- National Association of Pediatric Nurse Practitioners (NAPNAP)
- National Conference of Gerontological Nurse Practitioners
- National Organization of Nurse Practitioner Faculties (NONPF)
- American Academy of Nurse Practitioners (AANP)
- American College of Nurse Practitioners (ACNP)
- Nurse Practitioner Associates for Continuing Education (NPACE)
- National Association of School Nurses
- Association for Women's Health, Obstetrics, and Neonatal Nurses (AWHONN)
- The National Association of Nurse Practitioners in Women's Health (NPWH)

Healthy People 2000

A 1990 publication put out by the US Department of Health and Human Services, with another assessment in a 1995 publication. Follow-up on how it was going was in a December 1999 publication. There were 3 big objectives for the United States:
- Give Americans a longer, healthy lifespan.
- Lessen health problems for Americans.
- Give all Americans ways to get pre-emptive measures.

This publication had 300 particular aims founded upon 22 critical things that would give Americans communally and economically productive life spans. These aims centered upon giving everyone the same right to use, satisfactoriness, accessibility, stability, expenditure and value of medical attention. The aims were categorized into wide sections of well-being support, well-being safeguards and prevention. It included recognition of the main concerns of methodical compilation, investigation, understanding, distribution, and utilization of information to comprehend how our nation was doing health-wise and to plan successful ways to handle prevention. People, societies and groups had to take accountability for figuring out how these aims would come about before the year 2000.

Results:

In 1998/99, it was found that 15% of the aims of the project were accomplished for nutrition, mother and child wellness, heart disease, and mental wellness. It was going well in 8 out of 17 aims regarding mother and child wellness, including perinatal/infant mortality and doing assessments for fetal irregularities and hereditary problems. There was no success for 4 aims and no movement away for 5 aims of issues about fetal alcohol syndrome and low birth weight. 44% of aims were going well in areas that are linked to child immunizations, nursing babies, going to the dentist habitually, mammography assessments, and eating fruits and vegetables on a daily basis.

Healthy People 2010

Put out in the year 2000 by the US Department of Health and Human Services in order to do more with the goals that were originally put forth by Healthy Patients 2000. The goal was to do 2 things: give better quality and length to a patient's life and well-being and eradicate health inconsistencies. There are 467 aims under 28 main categories.

Goals:

Aims center around getting together for better health, getting rid of health irregularities, having more quality and length of well-being in life, and using technology for well-being. The aims are in groups, including: exercise, diet, smoking, instruction and society-founded plans, environmental well-being, stopping harm and aggression, work safety and well-being, dental well-being, getting to good health programs, family planning, mother-baby-child well-being, using medical paraphernalia safely, public health communications, well-being messages, prevention and staying healthy, cases of disability or secondary issues, heart disease and stroke, kidney disease, mental well-being and mental problems, respiratory irregularities, STDs, and drug/alcohol abuse. The 10 leading health indicators (LDH) include:

- Exercise
- Overweight/obese weight range
- Smoking/Drug and/or alcohol abuse
- Conscientious sexual activity
- Mental well-being/Harm and aggression
- Good atmosphere/Immunizations
- Being able to get to good medical attention

Patient consent

If you are doing research that has patients involved, the most vital piece to include is the assertion that everything will be private and confidential. This piece is necessary and it is against the law to leave it out.

Using new research

Use a new practice based on research in a clinical setting if the outcome of the research showed statistically significant results. It is hard in ambulatory care environment because the job is so challenging that there is not much time left for using new research. Lack of time is a factor in every medical care environment. Getting the research is not usually the problem since it can be acquired through the internet or in professional journals. Quite a bit of research has been done regarding ambulatory care environments. Using new research in a clinical setting commonly has the outcome of an alteration in the way things are done. Nursing is a lot like research.

Null hypothesis

There is no significant difference between the two groups.

Two-tailed *t* test

Compares 2 separate and individual groups with regard to a variable.

Four steps of research

Assess, plan, implement, and evaluate. These steps are much like what the nurse practitioner does when helping a patient.

Statistics

<u>Descriptive statistics:</u>
Utilized to depict a sample.

<u>Inferential statistics:</u>
Utilized when testing hypotheses

Types of data

Nominal level data is information such as ethnicity. Ordinal data is with regard to rank order (1st, 2nd, 3rd, etc.). Interval measurement examples include information with regard to calendar days, temperature, etc. Ratio measurement is often called true measurement; it is the only type that has units of measurement.

Martha Rogers

Debated that the creation of nurse practitioner as a position was a maneuver meant to trick nurses out of doing nursing and switch over to medicine, which would abate and undercut the nurse's particular role. It created a significant split in nursing and therefore made hindrances regarding the creation of nurse practitioner programs in institutions.

Note: clinical nurse specialist is one role that was made very easily with no major debate. Nurse practitioner, certified nurse midwife, and nurse anesthetist were all controversial.

Loretta Ford, RN, PhD, and Henry Silver, MD

Created the initial pediatric nurse practitioner program, which was located at the University of Colorado.

Mary Breckenridge

Began Frontier Nursing Service, located in underdeveloped rural mountains in Kentucky. This went on to include instruction for nurse midwives.

Agnes McGee

Offered the initial postgraduate program for nurse anesthetists. St. Vincent's Hospital, Portland, Oregon.

Hildegard Peplau

Began the initial psychiatric CNS program. Rutgers University.

Nurse practitioners

Policy expertise:

The most important is for the nurse practitioner to get political allies. Having political friends that can make decisions (i.e., in the legislature) lets the nurse practitioner contribute and stay up to date about issues.

Increasing NP abilities:

Three main areas that are vital for increasing what the nurse practitioner can do are writing prescriptions, reimbursement rights, and range of practice that is allowed under the law.

ICD-9-CM

International Classification of Diseases, 9th Edition; this has diagnostic codes that tell what medical problem, sickness, or harm the medical attention is for; utilized with billing insurance companies.

CPT

Current Procedural Terminology; these codes tell what procedure or medical attention was done; there are more than 7000. Both Medicare and state Medicaid carriers have to utilize these codes under the law.

HCPC

Health Care Financing Administration Common Procedure Coding System; this is utilized to make an account of supplies and medical tools.

Research variables

- Independent variable – Manipulated; the reason or the treatment.
- Dependent variable – Not controlled; result or outcome.
- Variate – How many variables there are.

Nursing theory

Every one includes person, health, and environment. Florence Nightingale began the way that nursing theory was done. Nursing theories are done in particular for nursing practice. Getting proof for abstract nursing theories is commonly impeded by having no way to sufficiently measure the concept. Nursing theory helps by giving a steady point of view of how to care for patients.

Betty Neuman

Found that there was a need for using new ideas with one or more of these: primary prevention, secondary prevention, and tertiary prevention.

Kurt Lewin

He put forth 3 ways to make alterations, including: unfreeze (change the way things have been done); move (create new reactions by using new data and altering the approach); refreeze (get to the new status quo, stabilize there, and use new actions along with the proper support so that the new way of doing things can be upheld).

Descriptive statistics

Summarizes, organizes, and simplifies the information in numerical form, as with mean, median, or mode.

- Mean – The average that is taken from a set of data.
- Median – The middle value, when all the data is lined up in order.
- Randomization – utilized so that there will be no bias in research. Used to get a good representation of the data.
- Multiple regression – Predicts values for one variable based on two or more other variables.
- Repeated measures t test – Statistical method; repeating the test, for example: pretest and posttest.
- Chi-square test – Statistical method of testing to determine the probability of getting the observed results by chance; uses a particular hypothesis.

Creation of nurse practitioner role

Not enough primary care doctors in the 1960s and 1970s because there was a trend toward having a medical specialty at that time. This caused a need for the nurse practitioner.

Understanding statistics:

It is important to be able to comprehend research that has been done to improve medical practices in a clinical setting. It is important for the reader to be able to read the data and comprehend how much worth the study has for his or her particular situation. Since the study might not give the complete scope of what was discovered and another person's analysis of it may be based on a particular point of view that is not relevant to the nurse, the nurse needs to be able to read and understand research reports. If the nurse reads a research report that does not include statistics, it still is not a frittered time because it could bring up new matter about best practices.

Pearson's correlation

Also called Pearson product-moment correlation coefficient (PMCC); common way to measure the relationship between two (or more) variables. It actually identifies the relationship.

Factor Analysis

Utilized for finding common elements between variables.

Qualitative nursing research

The aim is to find and describe concepts of nursing. It does not include exact measurements and does not generally include statistics.

Standard deviation

Measures the dispersion of data; it is the square root of variance.

Example: the regular ranges for blood work values would probably be put in a standard deviation as a statistic.

Steps to using research

- Find the problems
- Evaluate published work
- Create the new idea
- Assess
- Determine if you will use the new idea

Healthcare Practice

Might change if there is a radical difference and restructuring of how medical attention is given. Prior research done in hospitals might not be relevant any longer if the patient is not being treated in a hospital setting any longer.

Sample Scenarios

The initial medical attention required for an older woman with high cholesterol and irregular lipoprotein results.

In an elderly female patient with high cholesterol and irregular lipoprotein results, the proper course of treatment would be to begin a regimen of balanced nutrition and activity. Over time, she may need a bile acid sequestrate agent or estrogen replacement therapy if the nutrition and activity are not working. It is not necessary for the patient to see a cardiologist unless she presents with additional indications or when the medical attention and regimen of nutrition and activity are not working.

The initial drug to be given to a patient with chest pain, a blood pressure reading of 86/52 mm Hg, and indications of ischemia.

This patient needs to go to the ER, but as he is waiting for the ambulance, the nurse should give them acetylsalicylic acid (ASA), or aspirin. The dose is 81 mg PO. This will aid in stopping the development of platelet-aggregating elements and can stop a block in a coronary artery that has been constricted. Do not give this patient nitroglycerin if their blood pressure is less than 90 mm HG.

When dizziness as a symptom may be a sign of a heart problem.

If the patient says that the dizziness worsens when they stands up, it may be a heart problem, and might be a sign of significant cardiac dysrhythmias. When the patient is dizzy only in specific poses, it is a sign of non-life-threatening positional vertigo, a condition that is frequently seen in elderly patients. Dizziness that goes along with tinnitus (ringing in the ears) is frequently seen with significant labyrinthitis. If the patient also has quick breathing beforehand it could be a case of hyperventilation.

The initial step for a patient who has no history of coronary artery danger elements but presents with a cholesterol level of 255 mg/dL.

This patient should be checked again for cholesterol to find the HDL and LDL results prior to doing anything else. Finding these amounts aid in classifying the patients danger elements and help the nurse to know how much medical treatment is needed.

How to assess a fully grown man who has indications of coughing with blood, sweating during sleep, no problems with respiration or heart in the past, 97 beats per minute (bpm) pulse, 28 breaths per minute, 140/92 blood pressure and a temperature of 99°F with a thermometer.

For this patient, start by checking to see if he has tuberculosis (TB). Check for TB with a PPD test. Do a chest x-ray. Do sputum smear test to see if there is acid-fast bacillus. If the sputum smear is positive, it is a sign of TB and the patient will need medical help right away.

Tell the initial assessment that should be done for a patient presenting with shortness of breath.

When a patient presents with shortness of breath (dyspnea) the first thing to find out is what the patient is usually doing that brings on the problem. Ask whether it is a problem during action or inaction. Find out the amount of action that it takes to bring on the condition. This will help you to gauge how bad the problem actually is before taking further steps.

The HgbA$_{1c}$ assessment for a patient who has excessive urination and thirst and lessened body weight.

HgbA$_{1c}$ assessment – If it is more than 8.0%, the patient has not had good glucose management for several months prior to the assessment. The patient will require immediate medical attention if this assessment is greater than 8%.

The probable reason for hypercalcemia in a patient who is otherwise healthy with no signs of another condition.

High amounts of calcium in the blood is due to hyperparathyroidism in more than 60% of instances.

What to do if the patient does not have a patellar reflex.

This knee jerk occurs when a sharp tap is given to the patellar tendon. If there is no reaction, ask the patient to do Jendrassik's maneuver of flexing muscles that are not used in the patellar reflex test, and then do the reflex assessment again. Have the patient lock the two hands together with equal muscle contraction in the fingers. Compare the nonreaction of the first assessment to the reaction that is found when doing the Jendrassik maneuver.

How to handle a patient who comes in and says he has the worst headache he has ever had.

If the pain is not getting better with general over-the-counter medications, it is very important to make sure the patient is not experiencing a subarachnoid hemorrhage. Because the symptom of the worst headache ever is linked to this problem, the patient needs to go right away to see a neurologic surgeon.

When to medically handle a case of peptic ulcer disease (PUD) prior to doing any assessments.

This condition is linked to *Helicobacter pylori*. You can go ahead and begin medical attention before doing any assessments if the problem is alleviated with food, antacids, or throwing up. The pain that comes with this condition is generally experienced in the early hours of the day. If the pain is not consistent with this or if the condition also includes anemia or lessened body weight, you will need to do assessments to rule out another condition. If the indications go on after 2–3 months of medical attention, do endoscopy.

A possible diagnosis for when you feel a solid (but not sore) supraclavicular lymph node on the left side of someone's body.

This finding goes along with identifying thoracic or abdominal malignancy. It is a Virchow's node.

Who would be a sufficient candidate for urodynamic research?

A patient who has had problems with stress incontinence and urge incontinence, but has had no operation done for incontinence, would be a sufficient candidate.

What to do if someone has a mildly higher blood pressure, no prior high blood pressure problems, no ongoing conditions, and a high serum lab value (5.2 mg/dL).

The patient needs to see a nephrologist right away because the serum creatinine is getting close to the 6.0 mg/dL mark where dialysis is an option. In the meantime, do more lab tests so the nephrologist will have the results, including whole parathyroid hormone (PTH), liver function, lipid panel, renal panel, magnesium level, and calcium level. Doing these now will help the nephrologist identify what is making the patient suffer from renal failure. Also review what drugs the patient is taking to make sure there is nothing that is making renal failure occur such as an angiotensin-converting enzyme (ACE) inhibitor like Captopril. Get a good family medical history to make sure there is no hereditary kidney problem (e.g., Alport's syndrome).

What an assessment that shows a raised serum gonadotropin amount may indicate.

An indication of testicular disease. On the other hand, a raised prostate-specific antigen (PSA) indicates disease.

What assessments to do for a woman postmenopause who starts bleeding again.

When it starts after a year of having no period or goes on more than 6 months after starting HRT, do more assessments. A frequent reason for it is endometrial atrophy. Make an appointment for an endometrial biopsy. Also check other, more significant problems to make sure there is nothing more serious. The biopsy will help find the reason for the issue. Menopause is defined as finishing a year of amenorrhea after having the last period.

The proper medical attention for a patient that presents with digitalis toxic signs and is currently taking digitalis, potassium, theophylline, hydrochlorothiazide, and a calcium-channel blocker.

This condition is often linked to hypokalemia, so be sure to check for that. The signs include first-degree obstruction and cardiac aggravation that worsens over time. Find out all relevant information prior to changing the drugs that the patient is taking. Check the blood pressure and heart rate. Check the patient medications. Find out how much serum theophylline, digitalis, and potassium the patient is getting. If the potassium level is not high enough, this could be initiating a toxic outcome. Find out whether serum theophylline levels are inside of the scope of what is needed medically. Manage the blood pressure.

How to check a middle-age woman who has been taking a thiazide diuretic for a month for high blood pressure and came in to the office with cramping and dizziness.

For this woman, check the blood pressure, pulse, respirations, tenting, the condition/state of the skin, neck veins, STAT serum electrolytes, sodium, chloride, potassium, and STAT blood glucose. Thiazide diuretics stop sodium from being absorbed again and help sodium, chloride, and water come out. These drugs are used for treating hypertension. The extracellular fluid volume is lessened. The plasma- rennin action and aldosterone levels are heightened. This causes lessened potassium for the patient. Medical attention includes getting the volume back to normal with regular saline solution and managing the lack of potassium. When sodium levels are heightened too fast, unfixable neurological harm may occur.

Drugs used for lowering high blood pressure in a case where lifestyle management is ineffective.

If a diet low in salt, more activity, loss of body weight, and stopping smoking is not enough to lower the blood pressure, the patient will need to keep on the program of a healthier lifestyle and add a medication to help lower the blood pressure. Except when there is a reason that the drug is not a good idea, the drugs of choice are diuretics or beta-blockers (which are likely to lessen insulin sensitivity in the patient). If the case is not simple and no other conditions are present, the patient might need another type of medication, such as an ACE inhibitor instead of a beta-blocker (for someone with type 1 diabetes with proteinuria). Begin with a small amount of the medication in a long-acting form, once daily, and gradually increase or decrease the amount as needed.

Drugs used for lowering high blood pressure in an elderly patient.

If the patient is older, then a beta-blocker is not a good choice, because there is lessened beta-adrenergic receptor sensitivity for the elderly patient. Elderly patients need smaller amounts of calcium entry antagonists, ACE inhibitors, or diuretics. Too high a dose (in the elderly) will cause moodiness, impotence, weariness, and lessened ability to think clearly. Elderly patients are particularly prone to congestive heart failure and peripheral vascular insufficiency due to beta-adrenergic toxins.

What drug is best for an elderly patient with a new congestive heart failure case and high blood pressure?

Begin this patient on ACE inhibitors to start. This medication will keep the patient's renal function intact and not affect the patient's ability to have sexual relations as much as other medications. Make sure the potassium levels are checked. Watch renal function for alterations. An ACE inhibitor will not have as many adverse outcomes as other drugs.

What to do if a patient is taking an ACE inhibitor and gets a stubborn cough.

One adverse effect of ACE inhibitors is a stubborn cough. If the patient gets it, they can use an angiotensin-receptor blocker (ARB) as an alternative, but make sure the cough is not due to heart failure. When the patient has a severe renal inadequacy or if there is angioedema, the patient can use hydralazine/nitrate together. It is not a good idea to use antiarrhythmic agents, calcium-channel blockers, or nonsteroidal anti-inflammatory medications (NSAIDs).

The antimicrobial therapy choices for acute bronchitis that includes a secondary bacterial infection.

Antimicrobial therapy choices for acute bronchitis that includes a secondary bacterial infection:
- Erythromycin – 250–500 mg taken by mouth q.i.d. for 10 days if the patient has *Mycoplasma pneumoniae* or *Streptococcus pneumonia.*
- Amoxicillin – 250 mg taken by mouth t.i.d. for 10 days if the patient has *Streptococcus pneumoniae* or *Haemophilus influenzae.*
- Doxycycline – 100 mg b.i.d. for 10 days if the patient has chlamydia or *Mycoplasma pneumoniae.*
- Trimethoprim/sulfamethoxazole – 1 double-strength tablet taken by mouth b.i.d. for 10 days if the patient has *Haemophilus influenzae* or *Moraxella catarrhalis.*

The antimicrobial management choices for dealing with pneumonia that does not require hospitalization and is obtained from a community source.

Based on medical experience, antimicrobial management of pneumonia that is obtained through the community includes:
For patients who do not have another disease or condition:

- Erythromycin – 500 mg taken by mouth q.i.d., 14 days
- Clarithromycin – 250–500 mg taken by mouth b.i.d. 7–14 days
- Tetracycline – 500 mg taken by mouth q.i.d. 14 days, or doxycycline 100 mg b.i.d. 14 days if the patient cannot have macrolide.

If the patient does have another disease or condition:
- Cefuroxime axetil 250–500 mg taken by mouth b.i.d., 10 days
- Trimethoprim/sulfamethoxazole (TMP/SMX) – 160 mg TMP and 800 mg SMX taken by mouth b.i.d., 14 days (restricted employment of this drug; resistant *streptococcal pneumoniae*)
- Amoxicillin-potassium clavulanate – 500 mg taken by mouth b.i.d. or 875 mg b.i.d., 10 days
- Macrolides when the patient might have Legionnaire's disease
- Mixture treatment: amoxicillin-clavulanate in addition to macrolide or doxycycline
- Respiratory fluoroquinolone (for instance, levofloxacin)

The antimicrobial management choices for dealing with pneumonia that does require hospitalization and is obtained from a community source.

The antimicrobial management choices for dealing with pneumonia that was obtained in the hospital.

For pneumonia that was obtained in the community and needs hospitalization:
- Cefuroxime sodium 0.75–1.5 g given into the vein every 8 hours, 5–10 days.
- Ceftriaxone sodium – 1–2 g into the vein every 12–24 hours, 5–10 days.
- Macrolide into the vein when there could be Legionnaire's disease.
- Respiratory fluoroquinolone may be needed if the patient is not responding to a mixture of drugs.

If the patient has a case that was obtained in the hospital:
- Mixture treatment of antibiotics is necessary.
- Choose the drug based on the assumed organism.

The use of a beta-blocker for someone with ongoing respiratory complications.

This type of medication can cause more problems for someone with ongoing respiratory issues. Choose a different antihypertensive agent instead. A calcium-channel blocker may be used.

Give the initial treatment for a patient in a nursing home who has been in constant contact with someone who has TB.
What medication is needed for someone with ongoing airflow restriction that has seen more mucus coming out and has experienced problems with stuffiness?

Nursing home patient – Begin chemoprophylaxis right away and do skin assessment. If the test is negative, do it again in 3 months, but continue with chemoprophylaxis. After 3 months, you may discontinue the medication if the test is still negative.

Patient with airflow restriction – The patient will need to take an antibiotic if the mucus has become a different color (such as yellowish/green), thickness, or if there is more of it. They should not use a drug to stop coughing or an antihistamine.

The medical attention for a pregnant woman with hyperthyroidism.
How to alter a patient's insulin dose if they have low blood sugar each day at the same time that the regular insulin is peaking.

Hyperthyroidism – In the first trimester, use propylthiouracil. In the second trimester, use subtotal thyroidectomy and thyroid replacement.

Blood sugar – If the patient's blood sugar is low each day at the same time that the insulin is peaking, their insulin dose should be decreased.

Tell what drug is used for a type 2 diabetic that is having trouble maintaining a healthy weight.

If he is having trouble maintaining a healthy weight, metformin (Glucophage) may be used. This drug is linked to losing body weight and giving the patient less of a need to eat. The true reason for losing weight due to this drug is not currently understood. Metformin is counter indicated for a male with serum creatinine that is 1.5 mg/dL or more or 1.4 mg/dL in a female because that can give the patient a tendency for lactic acidosis. Lactic acidosis can be significant or deadly.

What medication to use for someone in her mid-30s who has hypothyroidism and raised TSH.

Normal TSH is 0.5–4.7 mU/L, so anything above that is considered higher than normal. The patient can be given a total replacement amount of levothyroxine (Synthroid), 0.1 mg PO qd. The drug might take 6 weeks to begin working, so assess the TSH after that much time has gone by. Using levothyroxine for a long time can cause significant osteoporosis, so be sure not to overuse this medication. Other side effects, which can be handled by stopping the medication for 3 days and beginning again with a smaller dose, include fast heart rate, inability to sleep, and perspiration. If there is chest pain, lower the dose, get an ECG, and see a doctor.

How to handle a patient who needs a bypass operation but also has hypothyroidism. The use of cold medications for a patient who is taking an antithyroid medication to handle hyperthyroidism.

Bypass and hypothyroidism – If the patient has minor to moderate hypothyroidism, they may still have a critical operation without danger if no previous replacement. Problems that could arise are not worse than problems that come up for patients who do not have hypothyroidism. Begin the replacement treatment after the operation to lower the danger to the heart.

Decongestants with antithyroid medication – The patient should stay away from the use of decongestants (like pseudoephedrine), which have sympathomimetics. The decongestant can cause unfavorable outcomes such as too much work for the central nervous system, fast and strong heartbeat, head pain, high blood pressure, anxiety, and more. Robitussin-CF or -PE may create fast and strong heartbeats and CNS overwork as well. The use of Robitussin-DM has a tendency for stomach problems, sleepiness, head pain, and skin irregularities.

What medication is needed for an older adult with an identification of hyperthyroidism that has had high blood pressure and a prior bypass operation?

Use levothyroxine (Synthroid), 0.025 mg every day for a time of 6 weeks. Raise the amounts slowly in 4–6 week increments pending getting to the needed amount. You cannot start with anything other than a small amount because too much medication could make the heart decompensate.

How to handle a patient who is putting out > 900 mg/day of uric acid.

This is found by looking at a 24-hour urine gathering. Prescribe allopurinol (Zyloprim) in an amount of 100 mg PO for a week. After that, raise it to up to 300 mg/day. This medication will lessen the serum uric acid. The aim is to get to < 6.5 mg/dL. Do not use aspirin, as it may cause gout.

The use of ibuprofen for an elderly patient.
The choice of methotrexate (Rheumatrex) in a patient with severe refractory rheumatoid arthritis (RA).

Ibuprofen – Some elderly patients are already dealing with lessened renal ability. Ibuprofen has the ability to make it even worse. This can cause nephrosis, cirrhosis, and congestive heart failure.

Methotrexate (Rheumatrex) for severe refractory RA – In each month that this drug is used, the patient needs to be checked for blood dyscrasias. Someone that is able to have children should not get pregnant while taking this medication.

How to handle a medical worker's instance of getting stuck with a needle.
A lab outcome that could cause one to consider HIV in the differential.

Needle stick – Put gloves on for protection, turn on running water, and bleed the area beneath the water for a few minutes. This is a better option than the use of an antiseptic on the skin.

HIV – Leukopenia and thrombocytopenia results could make HIV be part of the differential. An acute primary HIV infection makes there be less CD4 cells. This makes leukopenia and lessens the amount of platelets.

Note: the HIV infection gives the patient a significant and dangerous lessening of helper T-cells and more suppressor T-cells.

What to do for patient taking HIV medication and is feeling queasy, vomiting, and has stomach pain.

Do a CBC including differential, lipase, lactic acid, electrolytes, BUN, creatinine, and LFT assessments. It is not necessary to check how the immune system is working, as it will not alter how to handle the HIV or medication.

What medicine to use for a bee sting that is causing the patient to have trouble breathing.

Initial treatment should be epinephrine. For 1:1000, SC, use 0.3 to 0.5 mL/kg for a fully grown patient.

What medication can stop a patient who is taking NSAIDs from developing an ulcer?

To stop an ulcer from occurring, prescribe celecoxib (Celebrex).

How to handle *Helicobacter pylori* for someone with peptic ulcer disease (PUD).

For a fully grown patient, utilize these 3 together: clarithromycin (Biaxin), amoxicillin (Amoxil), and omeprazole (Prilosec).

How much TMP-SMX (Septra DS) needs to be used for a 75-year-old patient who has ongoing bacterial prostatitis.

For this patient, use one tablet b.i.d. for 30 days. It is advised to use it for a minimum of 30 days to keep the problem from coming back. Some patients will need ongoing suppression treatment for a longer duration of time.

How to help someone who chooses not to use hormone replacement therapy but is suffering with hot flashes.

Venlafaxine HCL (Effexor SR), which helps hot flashes (as seen in random-controlled trials). The dosage is 25–150 mg daily. Some patients think nonprescription or natural aids are less dangerous than prescriptions, but they can have adverse outcomes or they may interfere with other medications. Ask the patient about any other medications or natural supplements they may be taking.

Adding progesterone for a female who is already taking estrogen in postmenopause.

Taking it will give reduce a female patient's risk of developing endometrial cancer. A patient who has a uterus and is utilizing unopposed exogenous estrogen does have an increased chance of developing endometrial cancer, so it is a good idea to use progesterone to lessen the chance. Using it could make bleeding start, and a lot of females do not want that.

What medicine to use for a case of chancroid in a patient who is likely to be noncompliant.

Give Ceftriaxone (Rocephin), 250 mg IM, taken in one dose.

Tell how to check a patient who has one hand presenting as cool when compared with the other hand.

When one hand is cool when compared with the other, use the back of your fingers (because that is the area that can feel the best during examinations) to touch the lower arm and check how warm or cool it is, to determine how much of the patient's limb is presenting with poor circulation.

CPR Review/Cheat Sheet

Topic	New Guidelines
Conscious Choking	5 back blows, then 5 abdominal thrusts- adult/child
Unconscious Choking	5 chest compressions, look, 2 breaths-adult/child/infant
Rescue Breaths	Normal Breath given over 1 second until chest rises
Chest Compressions to Ventilation Ratios (Single Rescuer)	30:2 – Adult/Child/Infant
Chest Compressions to Ventilation Ratios (Two Rescuer)	30:2 – Adult 15:2 – Child/Infant
Chest Compression rate	About 100/minute – Adult/Child/Infant
Chest Compression Land marking Method	Simplified approach – center of the chest – Adult/Child 2 or 3 fingers, just below the nipple line at the center of the chest - Infant
AED	1 shock, then 2 minutes (or 5 cycles) of CPR
Anaphylaxis	Assist person with use of prescribed auto injector
Asthma	Assist person with use of prescribed inhaler

- Check the scene
- Check for responsiveness – ask, "Are you OK?"
- Adult - call 911, then administer CPR
- Child/Infant – administer CPR for 5 cycles, then call 911
- Open victim's airway and check for breathing – look, listen, and feel for 5 - 10 seconds
- Two rescue breaths should be given, 1 second each, and should produce a visible chest rise
- If the air does not go in, reposition and try 2 breaths again
- Check victim's pulse – chest compressions are recommended if an infant or child has a rate less than 60 per minute with signs of poor perfusion.
- Begin 30 compressions to 2 breaths at a rate of 1 breath every 5 seconds for Adult; 1 breath every 3 seconds for child/infant
- Continue 30:2 ratio until victim moves, AED is brought to the scene, or professional help arrives

AED

- ADULT/ Child over 8 years old - use Adult pads
- Child 1-8 years old – use Child pads or use Adult pads by placing one on the chest and one on the back of the child
- Infant under 1 year of age - AED not recommended

Pharmacology Generic/Trade Names of 50 Key Drugs in Medicine

1. Alprazolam — XANAX
2. Amitriptyline — ELAVIL
3. Amoxicillin/clavulanate potassium — AUGMENTIN
4. Betamethasone — CELESTONE
5. Bumetanide — BUMEX
6. Bupropion — WELLBUTRIN
7. Calcitriol — ROCALTROL
8. Ceforanide — PRECEF
9. Ceftazidime — FORTAZ
10. Cephalexin — KEFLEX
11. Ciprofloxacin — CIPRO
12. Clonazepam — KLONOPIN
13. Cyclobenzaprine — FLEXERIL
14. Diazepam — VALIUM
15. Dopamine — INTROPIN
16. Enalapril — VASOTEC
17. Eythromycin — E-MYCIN
18. Famotidine — PEPCID
19. Fluconazole — DiFLUCON
20. Fluoxetine — PROZAC
21. Furosemide — LASIX
22. Gentamicin — GARAMYCIN
23. Haloperidol — HALDOL
24. Hydroxyprogesterone caproate — DELALUTIN
25. Ibuprofen — MOTRIN
26. Ipratropium bromide — ATROVENT
27. Ketorolac — TORADOL
28. Lidocaine — XYLOCAINE
29. Lorazepam — ATIVAN
30. Meperidine — DEMEROL

31. Methicillin — STAPHCILLIN
32. Metoprolol — LOPRESSOR
33. Miconazole — MONISTAT
34. Nystatin — MYCOSTATIN
35. Omeprazole — PRILOSEC
36. Oxybutynin — DITROPAN
37. Oxymetholone — ANADROL
38. Pergolide — PERMAX
39. Phenytoin — DILANTIN
40. Prazepam — CENTRAX
41. Prednisone — DELTASONE
42. Procaine — NOVOCAIN
43. Promethazine — PHENERGAN
44. Propoxyphene — DARVON
45. Pseudoephedrine — SUDAFED
46. Silver sulfadiazine — SILVADENE
47. Temazepam — RESTORIL
48. Tolnaftate — TINACTIN
49. Vancomycin — VANCOCIN
50. Warfarin — COUMADIN

Special Report: What Your Test Score Will Tell You About Your IQ

Did you know that most standardized tests correlate very strongly with IQ? In fact, your general intelligence is a better predictor of your success than any other factor, and most tests intentionally measure this trait to some degree to ensure that those selected by the test are truly qualified for the test's purposes.

Before we can delve into the relation between your test score and IQ, I will first have to explain what exactly is IQ. Here's the formula:

Your IQ = 100 + (Number of standard deviations below or above the average)*15

Now, let's define standard deviations by using an example. If we have 5 people with 5 different heights, then first we calculate the average. Let's say the average was 65 inches. The standard deviation is the "average distance" away from the average of each of the members. It is a direct measure of variability - if the 5 people included Jackie Chan and Shaquille O'Neal, obviously there's a lot more variability in that group than a group of 5 sisters who are all within 6 inches in height of each other. The standard deviation uses a number to characterize the average range of difference within a group.

A convenient feature of most groups is that they have a "normal" distribution- makes sense that most things would be normal, right? Without getting into a bunch of statistical mumbo-jumbo, you just need to know that if you know the average of the group and the standard deviation, you can successfully predict someone's percentile rank in the group.

Confused? Let me give you an example. If instead of 5 people's heights, we had 100 people, we could figure out their rank in height JUST by knowing the average, standard deviation, and their height. We wouldn't need to know each person's height and manually rank them, we could just predict their rank based on three numbers.

What this means is that you can take your PERCENTILE rank that is often given with your test and relate this to your RELATIVE IQ of people taking the test - that is, your IQ relative to the people taking the test. Obviously, there's no way to know your actual IQ because the people taking a standardized test are usually not very good samples of the general population- many of those with extremely low IQ's never achieve a level of success or competency necessary to complete a typical standardized test. In fact, professional psychologists who measure IQ actually have to use non-written tests that can fairly measure the IQ of those not able to complete a traditional test.

The bottom line is to not take your test score too seriously, but it is fun to compute your "relative IQ" among the people who took the test with you. I've done the calculations below. Just look up your percentile rank in the left and then you'll see your "relative IQ" for your test in the right hand column-

Percentile Rank	Your Relative IQ	Percentile Rank	Your Relative IQ
99	135	59	103
98	131	58	103
97	128	57	103
96	126	56	102
95	125	55	102
94	123	54	102
93	122	53	101
92	121	52	101
91	120	51	100
90	119	50	100
89	118	49	100
88	118	48	99
87	117	47	99
86	116	46	98
85	116	45	98
84	115	44	98
83	114	43	97
82	114	42	97
81	113	41	97
80	113	40	96
79	112	39	96
78	112	38	95
77	111	37	95
76	111	36	95
75	110	35	94
74	110	34	94
73	109	33	93
72	109	32	93

71	108	31	93
70	108	30	92
69	107	29	92
68	107	28	91
67	107	27	91
66	106	26	90
65	106	25	90
64	105	24	89
63	105	23	89
62	105	22	88
61	104	21	88
60	104	20	87

Special Report: Retaking the Test

What Are Your Chances at Improving Your Score?

After going through the experience of taking a major test, many test takers feel that once is enough. The test usually comes during a period of transition in the test taker's life, and taking the test is only one of a series of important events. With so many distractions and conflicting recommendations, it may be difficult for a test taker to rationally determine whether or not he should retake the test after viewing his scores.

The importance of the test usually only adds to the burden of the retake decision. However, don't be swayed by emotion. There a few simple questions that you can ask yourself to guide you as you try to determine whether a retake would improve your score:

1. What went wrong? Why wasn't your score what you expected?

Can you point to a single factor or problem that you feel caused the low score? Were you sick on test day? Was there an emotional upheaval in your life that caused a distraction? Were you late for the test or not able to use the full time allotment? If you can point to any of these specific, individual problems, then a retake should definitely be considered.

2. Is there enough time to improve?

Many problems that may show up in your score report may take a lot of time for improvement. A deficiency in a particular math skill may require weeks or months of tutoring and studying to improve. If you have enough time to improve an identified weakness, then a retake should definitely be considered.

3. How will additional scores be used? Will a score average, highest score, or most recent score be used?

Different test scores may be handled completely differently. If you've taken the test multiple times, sometimes your highest score is used, sometimes your average score is computed and used, and sometimes your most recent score is used. Make sure you understand what method will be used to evaluate your scores, and use that to help you determine whether a retake should be considered.

4. Are my practice test scores significantly higher than my actual test score?

If you have taken a lot of practice tests and are consistently scoring at a much higher level than your actual test score, then you should consider a retake. However, if you've taken five practice tests and only one of your scores was higher than your actual test score, or if your practice test scores were only slightly higher than your actual test score, then it is unlikely that you will significantly increase your score.

5. Do I need perfect scores or will I be able to live with this score? Will this score still allow me to follow my dreams?

What kind of score is acceptable to you? Is your current score "good enough?" Do you have to have a certain score in order to pursue the future of your dreams? If you won't be happy with your current score, and there's no way that you could live with it, then you should consider a retake. However, don't get your hopes up. If you are looking for significant improvement, that may or may not be possible. But if you won't be happy otherwise, it is at least worth the effort.
Remember that there are other considerations. To achieve your dream, it is likely that your grades may also be taken into account. A great test score is usually not the only thing necessary to succeed. Make sure that you aren't overemphasizing the importance of a high test score.

Furthermore, a retake does not always result in a higher score. Some test takers will score lower on a retake, rather than higher. One study shows that one-fourth of test takers will achieve a significant improvement in test score, while one-sixth of test takers will actually show a decrease. While this shows that most test takers will improve, the majority will only improve their scores a little and a retake may not be worth the test taker's effort.

Finally, if a test is taken only once and is considered in the added context of good grades on the part of a test taker, the person reviewing the grades and scores may be tempted to assume that the test taker just had a bad day while taking the test, and may discount the low test score in favor of the high grades. But if the test is retaken and the scores are approximately the same, then the validity of the low scores are only confirmed. Therefore, a retake could actually hurt a test taker by definitely bracketing a test taker's score ability to a limited range.

Special Report: Test Anxiety

The very nature of tests caters to some level of anxiety, nervousness or tension, just as we feel for any important event that occurs in our lives. A little bit of anxiety or nervousness can be a good thing. It helps us with motivation, and makes achievement just that much sweeter. However, too much anxiety can be a problem; especially if it hinders our ability to function and perform.

"Test anxiety," is the term that refers to the emotional reactions that some test-takers experience when faced with a test or exam. Having a fear of testing and exams is based upon a rational fear, since the test-taker's performance can shape the course of an academic career. Nevertheless, experiencing excessive fear of examinations will only interfere with the test-takers ability to perform, and his/her chances to be successful.

There are a large variety of causes that can contribute to the development and sensation of test anxiety. These include, but are not limited to lack of performance and worrying about issues surrounding the test.

Lack of Preparation

Lack of preparation can be identified by the following behaviors or situations:

Not scheduling enough time to study, and therefore cramming the night before the test or exam
Managing time poorly, to create the sensation that there is not enough time to do everything
Failing to organize the text information in advance, so that the study material consists of the entire text and not simply the pertinent information
Poor overall studying habits

Worrying, on the other hand, can be related to both the test taker, or many other factors around him/her that will be affected by the results of the test. These include worrying about:

Previous performances on similar exams, or exams in general
How friends and other students are achieving
The negative consequences that will result from a poor grade or failure

There are three primary elements to test anxiety. Physical components, which involve the same typical bodily reactions as those to acute anxiety (to be discussed below). Emotional factors have to do with fear or panic. Mental or cognitive issues concerning attention spans and memory abilities.

Physical Signals

There are many different symptoms of test anxiety, and these are not limited to mental and emotional strain. Frequently there are a range of physical signals that will let a test taker know that he/she is suffering from test anxiety. These bodily changes can include the following:

Perspiring

Sweaty palms

Wet, trembling hands

Nausea

Dry mouth

A knot in the stomach

Headache

Faintness

Muscle tension

Aching shoulders, back and neck

Rapid heartbeat

Feeling too hot/cold

To recognize the sensation of test anxiety, a test-taker should monitor him/herself for the following sensations:

The physical distress symptoms as listed above

Emotional sensitivity, expressing emotional feelings such as the need to cry or laugh too much, or a sensation of anger or helplessness

A decreased ability to think, causing the test-taker to blank out or have racing thoughts that are hard to organize or control.

Though most students will feel some level of anxiety when faced with a test or exam, the majority can cope with that anxiety and maintain it at a manageable level. However, those who cannot are faced with a very real and very serious condition, which can and should be controlled for the immeasurable benefit of this sufferer.

Naturally, these sensations lead to negative results for the testing experience. The most common effects of test anxiety have to do with nervousness and mental blocking.

Nervousness

Nervousness can appear in several different levels:

The test-taker's difficulty, or even inability to read and understand the questions on the test
The difficulty or inability to organize thoughts to a coherent form
The difficulty or inability to recall key words and concepts relating to the testing questions (especially essays)
The receipt of poor grades on a test, though the test material was well known by the test taker

Conversely, a person may also experience mental blocking, which involves:

Blanking out on test questions
Only remembering the correct answers to the questions when the test has already finished.

Fortunately for test anxiety sufferers, beating these feelings, to a large degree, has to do with proper preparation. When a test taker has a feeling of preparedness, then anxiety will be dramatically lessened.

The first step to resolving anxiety issues is to distinguish which of the two types of anxiety are being suffered. If the anxiety is a direct result of a lack of preparation, this should be considered a normal reaction, and the anxiety level (as opposed to the test results) shouldn't be anything to worry about. However, if, when adequately prepared, the test-taker still panics, blanks out, or seems to overreact, this is not a fully rational reaction. While this can be considered normal too, there are many ways to combat and overcome these effects.

Remember that anxiety cannot be entirely eliminated, however, there are ways to minimize it, to make the anxiety easier to manage. Preparation is one of the best ways to minimize test anxiety. Therefore the following techniques are wise in order to best fight off any anxiety that may want to build.

To begin with, try to avoid cramming before a test, whenever it is possible. By trying to memorize an entire term's worth of information in one day, you'll be shocking your system, and not giving yourself a very good chance to absorb the information. This is an easy path to anxiety, so for those who suffer from test anxiety, cramming should not even be considered an option.

Instead of cramming, work throughout the semester to combine all of the material which is presented throughout the semester, and work on it gradually as the course goes by, making sure to master the main concepts first, leaving minor details for a week or so before the test.

To study for the upcoming exam, be sure to pose questions that may be on the examination, to gauge the ability to answer them by integrating the ideas from your texts, notes and lectures, as well as any supplementary readings.

If it is truly impossible to cover all of the information that was covered in that particular term, concentrate on the most important portions, that can be covered very well. Learn these concepts as best as possible, so that when the test comes, a goal can be made to use these concepts as presentations of your knowledge.

In addition to study habits, changes in attitude are critical to beating a struggle with test anxiety. In fact, an improvement of the perspective over the entire test-taking experience can actually help a test taker to enjoy studying and therefore improve the overall experience. Be certain not to overemphasize the significance of the grade - know that the result of the test is neither a reflection of self worth, nor is it a measure of intelligence; one grade will not predict a person's future success.

To improve an overall testing outlook, the following steps should be tried:

Keeping in mind that the most reasonable expectation for taking a test is to expect to try to demonstrate as much of what you know as you possibly can.

Reminding ourselves that a test is only one test; this is not the only one, and there will be others. The thought of thinking of oneself in an irrational, all-or-nothing term should be avoided at all costs.

A reward should be designated for after the test, so there's something to look forward to. Whether it be going to a movie, going out to eat, or simply visiting friends, schedule it in advance, and do it no matter what result is expected on the exam.

Test-takers should also keep in mind that the basics are some of the most important things, even beyond anti-anxiety techniques and studying. Never neglect the basic social, emotional and biological needs, in order to try to absorb information. In order to best achieve, these three factors must be held as just as important as the studying itself.

Study Steps

Remember the following important steps for studying:

Maintain healthy nutrition and exercise habits. Continue both your recreational activities and social pass times. These both contribute to your physical and emotional well being.

Be certain to get a good amount of sleep, especially the night before the test, because when you're overtired you are not able to perform to the best of your best ability.

Keep the studying pace to a moderate level by taking breaks when they are needed, and varying the work whenever possible, to keep the mind fresh instead of getting bored.

When enough studying has been done that all the material that can be learned has been learned, and the test taker is prepared for the test, stop studying and do something relaxing such as listening to music, watching a movie, or taking a warm bubble bath.

There are also many other techniques to minimize the uneasiness or apprehension that is experienced along with test anxiety before, during, or even after the examination. In fact, there are a great deal of things that can be done to stop anxiety from interfering with lifestyle and performance. Again, remember that anxiety will not be eliminated entirely, and it shouldn't be. Otherwise that "up" feeling for exams would not exist, and most of us depend on that sensation to perform better than usual. However, this anxiety has to be at a level that is manageable.

Of course, as we have just discussed, being prepared for the exam is half the battle right away. Attending all classes, finding out what knowledge will be expected on the exam, and knowing the exam schedules are easy steps to lowering anxiety. Keeping up with work will remove the need to cram, and efficient study habits will eliminate wasted time. Studying should be done in an ideal location for concentration, so that it is simple to become interested in the material and give it complete attention. A method such as SQ3R (Survey, Question, Read, Recite, Review) is a wonderful key to follow to make sure that the study habits are as effective as possible, especially in the case of learning from a textbook. Flashcards are great techniques for memorization. Learning to take good notes will mean that notes will be full of useful information, so that less sifting will need to be done to seek out what is pertinent for studying. Reviewing notes after class and then again on occasion will keep the information fresh in the mind. From notes that have been taken summary sheets and outlines can be made for simpler reviewing.

A study group can also be a very motivational and helpful place to study, as there will be a sharing of ideas, all of the minds can work together, to make sure that everyone understands, and the studying will be made more interesting because it will be a social occasion.

Basically, though, as long as the test-taker remains organized and self confident, with efficient study habits, less time will need to be spent studying, and higher grades will be achieved.

To become self confident, there are many useful steps. The first of these is "self talk." It has been shown through extensive research, that self-talk for students who suffer from test anxiety, should be well monitored, in order to make sure that it contributes to self confidence as opposed to sinking the student. Frequently the self talk of test-anxious students is negative or self-defeating, thinking that everyone else is smarter and faster, that they always mess up, and that if they don't do well, they'll fail the entire course. It is important to decreasing anxiety that awareness is made of self talk. Try writing any negative self thoughts and then disputing them with a positive statement instead. Begin self-encouragement as though it was a friend speaking. Repeat positive statements to help reprogram the mind to believing in successes instead of failures.

Helpful Techniques

Other extremely helpful techniques include:

Self-visualization of doing well and reaching goals

While aiming for an "A" level of understanding, don't try to "overprotect" by setting your expectations lower. This will only convince the mind to stop studying in order to meet the lower expectations.

Don't make comparisons with the results or habits of other students. These are individual factors, and different things work for different people, causing different results.

Strive to become an expert in learning what works well, and what can be done in order to improve. Consider collecting this data in a journal.

Create rewards for after studying instead of doing things before studying that will only turn into avoidance behaviors.

Make a practice of relaxing - by using methods such as progressive relaxation, self-hypnosis, guided imagery, etc - in order to make relaxation an automatic sensation.

Work on creating a state of relaxed concentration so that concentrating will take on the focus of the mind, so that none will be wasted on worrying.

Take good care of the physical self by eating well and getting enough sleep.

Plan in time for exercise and stick to this plan.

Beyond these techniques, there are other methods to be used before, during and after the test that will help the test-taker perform well in addition to overcoming anxiety.

Before the exam comes the academic preparation. This involves establishing a study schedule and beginning at least one week before the actual date of the test. By doing this, the anxiety of not having enough time to study for the test will be automatically eliminated. Moreover, this will make the studying a much more effective experience, ensuring that the learning will be an easier process. This relieves much undue pressure on the test-taker.

Summary sheets, note cards, and flash cards with the main concepts and examples of these main concepts should be prepared in advance of the actual studying time. A topic should never be eliminated from this process. By omitting a topic because it isn't expected to be on the test is only setting up the test-taker for anxiety should it actually appear on the exam. Utilize the course syllabus for laying out the topics that should be studied. Carefully go over the notes that were made in class, paying special attention to any of the issues that the professor took special care to emphasize while lecturing in class. In the textbooks, use the chapter review, or if possible, the chapter tests, to begin your review.

It may even be possible to ask the instructor what information will be covered on the exam, or what the format of the exam will be (for example, multiple choice, essay, free form, true-false). Additionally, see if it is possible to find out how many questions will be on the test. If a review sheet or sample test has been offered by the professor, make good use of it, above anything else, for the preparation for the test. Another great resource for getting to know the examination is reviewing tests from previous semesters. Use these tests to review, and aim to achieve a 100% score on each of the possible topics. With a few exceptions, the goal that you set for yourself is the highest one that you will reach.

Take all of the questions that were assigned as homework, and rework them to any other possible course material. The more problems reworked, the more skill and confidence will form as a result. When forming the solution to a problem, write out each of the steps. Don't simply do head work. By doing as many steps on paper as possible, much clarification and therefore confidence will be formed. Do this with as many homework problems as possible, before checking the answers. By checking the answer after each problem, a reinforcement will exist, that will not be on the exam. Study situations should be as exam-like as possible, to prime the test-taker's system for the experience. By waiting to check the answers at the end, a psychological advantage will be formed, to decrease the stress factor.

Another fantastic reason for not cramming is the avoidance of confusion in concepts, especially when it comes to mathematics. 8-10 hours of study will become one hundred percent more effective if it is spread out over a week or at least several days, instead of doing it all in one sitting. Recognize that the human brain requires time in order to assimilate new material, so frequent breaks and a span of study time over several days will be much more beneficial.

Additionally, don't study right up until the point of the exam. Studying should stop a minimum of one hour before the exam begins. This allows the brain to rest and put things in their proper order. This will also provide the time to become as relaxed as possible when going into the examination room. The test-taker will also have time to eat well and eat sensibly. Know that the brain needs food as much as the rest of the body. With enough food and enough sleep, as well as a relaxed attitude, the body and the mind are primed for success.

Avoid any anxious classmates who are talking about the exam. These students only spread anxiety, and are not worth sharing the anxious sentimentalities.

Before the test also involves creating a positive attitude, so mental preparation should also be a point of concentration. There are many keys to creating a positive attitude. Should fears become rushing in, make a visualization of taking the exam, doing well, and seeing an A written on the paper. Write out a list of affirmations that will bring a feeling of confidence, such as "I am doing well in my English class," "I studied well and know my material," "I enjoy this class." Even if the affirmations aren't believed at first, it sends a positive message to the subconscious which will result in an alteration of the overall belief system, which is the system that creates reality.

If a sensation of panic begins, work with the fear and imagine the very worst! Work through the entire scenario of not passing the test, failing the entire course, and dropping out of school, followed by not getting a job, and pushing a shopping cart through the dark alley where you'll live. This will place things into perspective! Then, practice deep breathing and create a visualization of the opposite situation - achieving an "A" on the exam, passing the entire course, receiving the degree at a graduation ceremony.

On the day of the test, there are many things to be done to ensure the best results, as well as the most calm outlook. The following stages are suggested in order to maximize test-taking potential:

Begin the examination day with a moderate breakfast, and avoid any coffee or beverages with caffeine if the test taker is prone to jitters. Even people who are used to managing caffeine can feel jittery or light-headed when it is taken on a test day.
Attempt to do something that is relaxing before the examination begins. As last minute cramming clouds the mastering of overall concepts, it is better to use this time to create a calming outlook.

Be certain to arrive at the test location well in advance, in order to provide time to select a location that is away from doors, windows and other distractions, as well as giving enough time to relax before the test begins.

Keep away from anxiety generating classmates who will upset the sensation of stability and relaxation that is being attempted before the exam.

Should the waiting period before the exam begins cause anxiety, create a self-distraction by reading a light magazine or something else that is relaxing and simple.

During the exam itself, read the entire exam from beginning to end, and find out how much time should be allotted to each individual problem. Once writing the exam, should more time be taken for a problem, it should be abandoned, in order to begin another problem. If there is time at the end, the unfinished problem can always be returned to and completed.

Read the instructions very carefully - twice - so that unpleasant surprises won't follow during or after the exam has ended.

When writing the exam, pretend that the situation is actually simply the completion of homework within a library, or at home. This will assist in forming a relaxed atmosphere, and will allow the brain extra focus for the complex thinking function.

Begin the exam with all of the questions with which the most confidence is felt. This will build the confidence level regarding the entire exam and will begin a quality momentum. This will also create encouragement for trying the problems where uncertainty resides.

Going with the "gut instinct" is always the way to go when solving a problem. Second guessing should be avoided at all costs. Have confidence in the ability to do well.

For essay questions, create an outline in advance that will keep the mind organized and make certain that all of the points are remembered. For multiple choice, read every answer, even if the correct one has been spotted - a better one may exist.

Continue at a pace that is reasonable and not rushed, in order to be able to work carefully. Provide enough time to go over the answers at the end, to check for small errors that can be corrected.

Should a feeling of panic begin, breathe deeply, and think of the feeling of the body releasing sand through its pores. Visualize a calm, peaceful place, and include all of the sights, sounds and sensations of this image. Continue the deep breathing, and take a few minutes to continue this with closed eyes. When all is well again, return to the test.

If a "blanking" occurs for a certain question, skip it and move on to the next question. There will be time to return to the other question later. Get everything done that can be done, first, to guarantee all the grades that can be compiled, and to build all of the confidence possible. Then return to the weaker questions to build the marks from there.

Remember, one's own reality can be created, so as long as the belief is there, success will follow. And remember: anxiety can happen later, right now, there's an exam to be written!

After the examination is complete, whether there is a feeling for a good grade or a bad grade, don't dwell on the exam, and be certain to follow through on the reward that was promised...and enjoy it! Don't dwell on any mistakes that have been made, as there is nothing that can be done at this point anyway.

Additionally, don't begin to study for the next test right away. Do something relaxing for a while, and let the mind relax and prepare itself to begin absorbing information again.

From the results of the exam - both the grade and the entire experience, be certain to learn from what has gone on. Perfect studying habits and work some more on confidence in order to make the next examination experience even better than the last one.

Learn to avoid places where openings occurred for laziness, procrastination and day dreaming.

Use the time between this exam and the next one to better learn to relax, even learning to relax on cue, so that any anxiety can be controlled during the next exam. Learn how to relax the body. Slouch in your chair if that helps. Tighten and then relax all of the different muscle groups, one group at a time, beginning with the feet and then working all the way up to the neck and face. This will ultimately relax the muscles more than they were to begin with. Learn how to breathe deeply and comfortably, and focus on this breathing going in and out as a relaxing thought. With every exhale, repeat the word "relax."

As common as test anxiety is, it is very possible to overcome it. Make yourself one of the test-takers who overcome this frustrating hindrance.

Special Report: Additional Bonus Material

Due to our efforts to try to keep this book to a manageable length, we've created a link that will give you access to all of your additional bonus material.

Please visit http://www.mo-media.com/np/bonuses to access the information.